D1521382

Fertile vs. Infertile

---

*How infections affect your fertility
and your baby's health*

---

by Attila Toth, M.D.

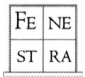

FE NE
ST RA

Fertile vs. Infertile: How infections affect your fertility and your baby's health

Published by Fenestra Books™
610 East Delano Street, Suite 104, Tucson, Arizona 85705 U.S.A.
www.fenestrabooks.com

Publisher's Cataloguing-in-Publication

Toth, A.
    Fertile vs. infertile : how infections affect your
fertility and your baby's health / by Attila Toth.
        p. cm.
    Includes bibliographical references.
    LCCN 2004104784
    ISBN 1587363321 (hardc.)
    ISBN 1587363879 (paperb.)

    1. Infertility--Popular works. 2. Infertility--
Chemotherapy. 3. Antibiotics. I. Title.

RC889.T678 2004   616.6'92061
                            QBI04-200273

ACKNOWLEDGEMENT

I am grateful to Jack Maguire for helping in the writing and editing of this book. His feedback as a layperson was invaluable.

I dedicate this book to all my patients, who have inspired me to write this book; their fascinating histories helped to illustrate the text.

RECOMMENDATION

I recommend this book to young and old alike. If you are not yet ready to start a family, you will find this book an invaluable tool for future planning. If you are in the midst trying to have a family, the book will help you navigate through reproduction with the optimal possible outcome. If all that is behind you, in reading these pages you will understand why things worked out the way they did—why you never had children or if you had them, why they turned out the way they did.

TABLE OF CONTENTS

PREFACE

Being unable to produce a much-wanted child is a singularly heartbreaking experience. It seems not only unfair but also unnatural. In fact, the feeling that it is somehow unnatural is not far from the truth. Left to themselves, the male and female reproductive systems are hardy and well engineered to succeed. When they do fail, it's almost always because of outside invaders: bacteria and other infectious agents (collectively called pathogens) that wreak critical damage on vital body tissues and mechanisms.

The good news is that proper antibiotic treatment—the safest, least invasive, and least costly form of infertility treatment—can usually restore fertility. The bad news is that antibiotic treatment is often bypassed in favor of the quick technological fix, which involves more expensive and risky but more impressively sophisticated procedures like hormone therapy, in vitro (or test tube) fertilization, and intrauterine insemination.

This book is a wake-up call to people suffering from infertility and the doctors who treat them. It makes the case for returning to basic common sense in treating infertility. It spells out exactly why we need to pay more attention to the biggest troublemakers in infertility cases—pathogens—and the most potentially effective infertility treatment—antibiotic therapy.

My previous book, *The Fertility Solution*, sounded this call 12 years ago. Since then, amazing progress has been made in appreciating the pathogenic sources of infertility and, as a result, in administering proper antibiotic treatment. However, recent discoveries have made the need to focus on these issues increasingly more urgent.

Over the past decade, a vast amount of evidence has been accumulated to show that pathogens are passed not only from one sexual partner to the other in reproductive fluids, but also from mother to child in fluids associated with a contaminated uterus or birth canal. Meanwhile, an even more startling picture has been developing from scientific research: Pathogens have been shown to trigger damage leading not only to infertility, but also to a growing list of other major health problems, including different forms of heart disease, cancer, and immune-related illnesses. Many of these illnesses were, and still are, commonly attributed to genetic or environmental factors, but such notions are now being challenged on every front as scientific research continues to uncover more about pathogens and their astonishing capabilities.

In this book, I offer evidence from my own long and extensive clinical experience to demonstrate that pathogens are major causes of infertility as well as many other health problems. I also describe in detail how antibiotic therapy can restore fertility and help guarantee better overall health for you, your child, and even your child's descendents. Finally, I give you specially designed questionnaires that you can use to estimate how seriously you may be threatened by infertility and other significant diseases.

Throughout the book, I cite an abundance of scientific research that supports my claims about pathogens and their connection to infertility and a host of major illnesses. Regrettably, there is no comprehensive study that absolutely confirms all of these claims. The scope of such a study is well beyond the capabilities of a single research team or clinic. Most likely the proof will have to emerge out of the collective contribution of hundreds of researchers and clinics. I hope the book can stimulate public and private agencies to devote more time, energy, and resources to this crucially important work.

Even more, I hope the book can help individual couples in their personal struggle to overcome infertility and create the healthy baby they yearn to bring into the world. The future of all of us is at stake.

CHAPTER 1

PLANNING FOR THE BEST POSSIBLE BABY

In all our deliberations, we must be mindful of the impact of our decision on the seven generations to follow.
—*Great Laws of the Six Nation Iroquois Confederacy*

Bringing a child into the world is one of the most amazing and fulfilling experiences a human being can have. In keeping with this wonder, it is also among nature's most miraculous events.

Modern science has made many noteworthy advances in overriding infertility problems to produce a child. In addition to hormone therapy and various kinds of corrective surgery, we have the more complex strategies collectively labeled "assisted reproduction technology" or ART. They include in vitro fertilization (or "test tube" conception), intrauterine insemination (injecting sperm into the uterus), intratubal insemination (injecting sperm into the fallopian tubes) and other highly sophisticated procedures designed to jump-start the mysterious chain of circumstances that leads to a new life. But these are only shots in the dark.

In actual practice, fewer than 30 percent of ART procedures result in a birth, according to the most recent data published by the Center for Disease Control (CDC), based on annual reports of the

American Society for Reproductive Medicine (ASRM) and the Society of Assisted Reproductive Technology (SART) for years 1999 and 2000 [1,2]. For women over age 30, the percentage drops even lower year by year.

Other adverse factors also need to be noted. An ART-assisted birth is more likely to produce a baby with low birth weight, a condition that can have a profoundly negative influence on the lifelong health of the child [3]. An article in the March 2002 edition of the New England Journal of Medicine categorized this risk as "significant" [4]. The mother involved in an ART-assisted birth is also exposed to an elevated risk of health problems. The 2002 edition of the medical journal Human Reproduction revealed that women who underwent ART were twice as likely to develop preeclampsia [5]. A potentially life-threatening condition associated with pregnancy, preeclampsia can feature elevated blood pressure, swelling of brain tissue, defective blood coagulation, organ damage, and, in its most severe form, a collapse of the circulatory system. A woman who conceives through ART, especially if she is beyond her mid-thirties, is also more likely to deliver after an abnormal labor process, often resulting in cesarean section [6].

The possibility of additional complications in the pregnancy or in the well-being of the child or the mother is also greater in ART cases than in ones that rely on other, less technological forms of treatment [7-11]. I'll return to these issues in the chapters to come. For now, the important point to keep in mind is that ART may be a remarkable medical achievement, but it is also a dangerous proposition. Unfortunately, many infertility specialists and centers tend to short-circuit due consideration of safer and possibly more effective therapies by channeling patients to ART too quickly.

Despite all of our medical expertise, we still don't know exactly why and how a new life starts or, in many cases, fails to begin. Nor can we be sure of the result when we seek to assist or even force the process by artificial means. Instead of achieving our desired objective—a healthy baby—by utilizing ART, we could easily wind up worsening our reproductive potential or creating one or more babies with severely compromised health.

As a physician, I have a deep love for and commitment to science, but my reverence for nature is even greater. In this era when so many people rush to solve their reproductive problems with ART, it's important to remember that science knows much less about childbirth than most of us think. While ART can provide options in the attempt to overcome infertility—each of which I've offered patients myself—its proper place remains as a last resort, and then only after a great deal of research and soul-searching regarding the possible consequences. It's a decision-making challenge that we'll investigate later in the book.

First and foremost in our efforts to give birth, we need to respect nature as much as we can and move step-by-step with great care and responsibility. Not only are we dealing with one of nature's most awesome miracles, but another vital issue is also at stake. Assuming a child is born, his or her health at birth is likely to affect the health of his or her descendants for generations to come, as the chapters ahead will clarify.

For both of these reasons, and for the greater happiness and welfare of all parties immediately involved, it's in the best interest of every prospective parent to aim for producing the healthiest possible baby in the healthiest possible manner. The main purpose of this book is to assist you in realizing this worthiest of all goals.

INFERTILITY: AN EPIDEMIC IN THE MAKING

The fact that you are reading these words probably means that you are now going through one of life's most heart-wrenching experiences: trying unsuccessfully to produce a child. Maybe you've been plagued by a long history of infertility, giving you vivid images to add to your fear this time around. Perhaps you're engaged in your first attempt to conceive, and, not being able to do so, you're lost in the terrifying dark. Possibly you suspect that you or your partner's current age, physical condition, or lifestyle is operating against you.

Whatever your situation, I can understand and empathize. Even more important, I can help. This book will help guide you through the often baffling mysteries of infertility and its treatments. It will also enable you to choose and negotiate the best possible treatment program with your doctor and other professionals in the field.

For over twenty-five years, I have practiced as a pathologist and obstetrician-gynecologist in New York City, treating or consulting in the treatment of over fifty thousand individuals and couples experiencing infertility. When I was the first physician in the treatment of an infertile couple, sixty percent of them have managed to have babies, a success rate far greater than the norm. I'm convinced that this happy outcome results from always taking the most logical, compassionate, and least invasive approach to each case of infertility. First, we thoroughly address all potential sources of a couple's reproductive problems. Then we do everything possible to restore that couple's natural reproductive capability before moving on, if desired, to more complicated and risky strategies for overriding the problems. Specifically, I focus right from the beginning on the major role that bacteria, viruses, and other infectious agents (collectively called "pathogens") can play in causing infertility.

Throughout my career, I've specialized in the field of pathogens. During that same time period in society at large, there's been a dramatic increase in both the infertility rate and in scientific discoveries connecting pathogens more directly to a broad spectrum of illnesses, diseases, and adverse medical conditions. In this book, you'll see how these two developments can be related, and what effect this connection can have on your ability to produce a baby.

Experts agree that the past few decades have brought an epidemic of infertility. The most recent report of the National Center for Health Statistics states that the percentage of women who have never given birth by age 40 has risen by more than half in approximately 30 years: from 10.6 in 1970 to 16.5 in 1995 (statistics after 1995 are unavailable). This increase is startling, even allowing for the ever-greater number of women who choose to remain childless or who postpone attempts to conceive a child until later in life [12, 13].

For women age 40 or older, the actual number of births has always been much smaller than the number of births in lower age categories. According to a 2001 report released by the Centers for Disease Control, the average 20-year-old woman has a 9 percent risk of infertility. This percentage doubles by age 35 and then doubles again, to 36 percent, by age 40. By age 43, a woman has an infertility risk of 70 percent [14].

Even more startling, the figures given in the report for the past three decades reflect a comparable year-by-year rise in infertility risk for each age group. This means that despite their growing reliance on more and more sophisticated high-tech therapies, women in every category, and especially women over age 40, have been steadily losing ground for almost 30 years in their efforts to have a child.

It is commonly said in the media and, regrettably, in many doctors' offices that the average woman over 40 simply has biology against her. However, as this book will clarify, the problem is often not a "natural" deterioration of reproductive capability but a longstanding, far advanced infection—one that can be eradicated with proper antibiotic treatment, given timely administration. It's welcome news to many women in this age group who are understandably panicked by the grim verdict routinely cast on their chances to bear children, especially if they've felt compelled to put off childbearing during their twenties and thirties in order to build a career. The truth is that they are by nature far more capable of bearing children than current statistics indicate, provided their reproductive systems remain protected from infection.

Meanwhile, as the infertility rate has continued to rise higher and higher with each passing year, science has made more and more significant discoveries linking pathogens like bacteria and viruses to serious illnesses. Among them are infertility, heart disease, high blood pressure, various cancers (such as breast, prostate, cervical, and liver), diabetes, hepatitis C, stomach ulcers, pulmonary hypertension, and complex "new" disease assisting conditions like Acquired Immune Deficiency Syndrome (AIDS).

At the end of the last millennium, a cover article in Natural History magazine summarized the prevailing wisdom on this matter:

> In the past three decades, research has increasingly implicated infection as a cause of diseases that many still think of as produced solely by lifestyle factors (stress, diet, lack of exercise), environmental pollution, or genetic inheritance. Between 15 and 20 percent of all human cancers are now attributed to infection. A bacterium—Helicobacter pylori—has been implicated as the cause of peptic ulcers and is also connected to stomach cancer. In heart disease, evidence that the stage is set by the bacterium Chlamydia pneumoniae looks stronger and stronger every month. In short, we seem to be in the middle, not at the end, of our effort to comprehend the scope of infectious diseases [15].

As we look back over all the relevant research accumulated since 1970, much of which is referenced in this book, it becomes obvious that the more insidious, complicated, and mysterious a health problem appears to be, the more likely it is that infectious agents may be at least partially responsible. In the vast majority of cases, infertility qualifies as this kind of perplexing health problem. And, as you will discover in these pages, so do many other common and uncommon illnesses that may very well have an impact on either a man's or a woman's ability to conceive.

Overall, it is estimated that 10 to 15 percent of American couples in their reproductive years suffer from infertility [16]. From a biological perspective, this figure is too large to make sense. If left to nature, infertility weeds itself out from generation to generation long before the rate of infertility in any one generation gets anywhere near that high.

To make matters worse, the true percentage of infertile couples today is probably much bigger. Besides the couples that actually report having problems, there are, no doubt, many "cryptic" cases. Among them are individuals or partners who don't report their infertility; those who choose not to have children and, therefore, are unaware of their infertility; and those who have only one child and, knowingly or not, suffer secondary infertility: the inability to have additional children [17].

The only explanation for an infertility rate so far out of proportion with logic and nature is that some specific agent or combination of agents is "breeding" infertility among us, and this breeding process is increasing from generation to generation. It is my firm belief, as well as my clinical experience, that the culprits are pathogens, and I share this conviction with an ever-growing number of other doctors and scientists. Other factors may also be involved in a particular case of infertility, but, as this book will explain, infectious agents clearly merit our full attention.

HOW DO WE DEFINE "INFERTILITY"?

In most medical sources, including reports from the National Centers for Disease Control and Prevention, infertility is defined as the failure to achieve conception after at least one year of unprotected intercourse with reasonable frequency (two to three times a week). I believe this definition is too conservative. As a result, it no doubt keeps many cases of possible infertility from being identified at an earlier stage, when treatment can often be more effective.

Assuming both partners have clean, healthy, intact reproductive systems, there is no biological reason why they shouldn't achieve conception in three months. Any longer period of time before conceiving suggests an infertile—or, as some experts prefer, sub-fertile—condition.

In addition, I don't think that the standard definition of infertility extends far enough into the reproductive process. I believe that the proper definition should encompass not just getting pregnant, but also having a good pregnancy and birth. This means the prospective mother should come to term within a few days of her due date, without medical intervention, and deliver the baby spontaneously, not by means of induced labor or cesarean section. The birth should entail no injury or infectious complications for the mother or the baby. Finally, the baby should be in good health.

What constitutes a "healthy" baby, beyond the lack of obvious physical defects or problems in functioning? This issue is one of the most critical in medical science, in human history, and in family planning. And yet, it is one of the least understood and appreciated, perhaps because it involves acknowledging truths that are often difficult to face.

The first and most prevalent sign of an unhealthy child is less-than-average size, even during the pregnancy itself. Other post-birth indicators are colic and slowness or other complications in physical, mental, or emotional development.

Also included among the symptoms of poor health are repeated bouts of infection-related illnesses, such as tonsillitis, ear infections, and bronchial asthma. Even a healthy child can experience occasional, short-term illnesses of this nature, usually after contact with an infected playmate. The hallmark of a sickly child is recurring infections readily triggered by the slightest environmental changes and often unattributable to any particular contact or event.

Additional congenital health problems may not become apparent until the child's school years or even later. In the 2002 edition of *Southern Medical Journal*, Drs. York and Devoe report ample evidence that low birth weight infants, beside exhibiting a host of other medical problems, go on to develop complex learning disorders and to exhibit poor performance in arithmetic and verbal functioning. Specifically, studies summarized in the article reveal that up to 45 percent of low birth weight babies had learning problems compared to 14 percent of normal weight babies; and seven percent in the former category wound up in special education versus only one percent in the latter. Other, possibly related problems that have been linked to low birth weight include a significantly greater-than-average tendency toward depression, inattention (including attention-deficit disorder), passiveness, restlessness, anti-social behavior, and low IQ scores [18].

In my experience with patients, a baby's low birth weight—as well as many of the other problems cited above, whether or not the birth weight was low—can most often be linked to an infected uterine environment. This fact adds to my conviction that the first nine (or fewer) months that we live in the uterus have a far more significant effect on everything we become as human beings than all of the years we live after birth.

In cases of conception and birth after the uterine environment has been restored to health by comprehensive antibiotic therapy, the results have almost always been unilaterally positive: an uncomplicated pregnancy, a trouble-free delivery within a few days of the projected due date, and, most gratifying of all, a normal-weight baby who exhibits none of the abnormal physical, mental, or emotional problems cited above. When I first interview people who come to my clinic, anything short of this positive scenario in their prior reproductive history sends up a warning signal of possible infection-related infertility.

The most critical reason to expand our understanding of what constitutes infertility is to allow for the earliest and therefore most effective possible treatment. Unfortunately, in cases of reproductive difficulty where pathogens are involved—and I believe they are implicated in the majority of situations—a sad truth prevails: the longer the condition exists, the stronger it grows and the more likely it is to leave behind irreparable damage. For infertile couples whose infections go untreated, this translates into an ever-escalating risk that they won't be able to conceive, that the prospective mothers will suffer complications during pregnancy, or that the health of the baby (assuming birth occurs) will be compromised.

WHAT CAUSES INFERTILITY?

As I've already mentioned, my experience and research tell me that pathogens play a major or contributing role in most cases of infertility. Frequently they help to cause or aggravate one of the more obvious conditions listed below. However, they can also be solely responsible for an individual's or a couple's inability to produce a baby. Once a pathogen settles into human tissue, it can initiate all sorts of harmful swelling, blocking, and scarring, much of which can lead to more advanced conditions that are more easily identifiable.

In the next section of this chapter, we'll look at how pathogens get transmitted into your reproductive system. First, let's consider the diagnoses that are most commonly associated with infertility.

Women:

Among women, infertility is generally associated with one or more of the following conditions, beginning with the most common (see figures 3 and 4 [pages 52 and 54] for anatomical references):

- Damaged fallopian tubes: Because the fallopian tubes are blocked, scarred, or otherwise dysfunctional, the sperm is unable to unite with the egg or the united pair are unable to descend to the uterus (which can lead to an ectopic pregnancy).

- Abnormal ovulation: Because of hormonal deficiencies or imbalances, egg production is not functioning as it should.

- Pelvic Inflammatory Disease (PID): A catch-all term applied to any inflammation of one or more of the pelvic organs, including those involved in reproduction, that prevents or complicates either a conception or a pregnancy.

- Endometriosis: During menstruation, segments of the uterine lining are washed into the abdominal cavity and form scar tissue (adhesions).

- Damaged ovaries: Scarring of the ovaries hinders or precludes normal egg development or release.

- Luteal phase defect: After the ovulatory phase of menstruation, there is a delay in the proper development of the uterine lining due to inadequate hormone production or the lining's inability to respond to normal hormone levels.

- Hostile cervical mucus: The cervix (located between the vagina and the uterus) harbors excessive acid introduced by infection and/or antibodies formed against infection. Either the acid or the antibodies can kill sperm cells before they're able to reach the eggs for fertilization.

- Incidental causes: The reproductive system is somehow damaged as the result of a neighboring abdominal disease, a tumor (fibroid or otherwise), surgery, therapy (such as chemotherapy), drug exposure, or physical trauma.

- Immunological causes: Anywhere in the woman's reproductive system, antibodies formed in response to previous contaminations by bacterial, viral, or other infectious agents attack the reproductive cells.

MEN

Among men, infertility is most often linked with one or more of the following conditions, beginning with the most common (see figure 3 [page 53] for anatomical reference):

- Idiopathic low sperm count: For unknown reasons, but probably due to complications in their prenatal development, the testes are incapable of producing sufficient sperm to ensure fertilization.

- Dilated veins around the testicles (varicocele): Enlarged veins raise the temperature in the scrotum, resulting in fewer and malformed or malfunctioning sperm.

- Damaged sperm ducts: The sperm ducts (also known as vas deferens and epididymis) are blocked, scarred, or congenitally missing, which prevents the sperm from reaching the seminal fluid.

- Inflammation can affect any part of the reproductive tract with adverse consequences (urethra, prostate, seminal vesicles, epididymis, or testes).

- Hormone deficiency: There is an insufficiency or imbalance in the release of the pituitary hormones which stimulate sperm production.

- Impotence: One or more causes render the man incapable of erection and ejaculation inside the vagina. They include: disease (such as hardening of the arteries, high blood pressure, diabetes, or kidney disease); environmental factors (such as medication regimens or substance abuse); trauma (such as spinal cord injury), and psychological conditions (such as performance anxiety or premature ejaculation).

- Incidental causes: The reproductive system is somehow damaged as the result of a neighboring abdominal disease, a tumor, surgery, therapy (such as chemotherapy), drug exposure, or physical trauma.

We'll examine each of these causes in detail, as well as the various strategies for preventing, treating, or overcoming them, in Chapters 3 through 6.

How Are Damaging Infections Transmitted?

Because pathogens are so often implicated in a couple's infertility, it is important to know how they get transmitted. As you will learn in the chapters to come, this knowledge can help you, the prospective parent, to safeguard not only your own health—reproductive and otherwise—but also the health of your baby and his or her descendants.

Essentially, damaging bacteria, viruses, and other infectious agents are transmitted from person to person in two ways: horizontally and vertically. Let's consider each one separately.

Horizontal transmission involves one sex partner infecting the other through the exchange of contaminated body fluids. Sometimes infecting partners know that they carry one or more pathogens, but most often they don't. Perhaps they have no physical symptoms—such as pain, fever, or abnormal fluid discharge from the genitals—to suggest to them that they may be infected. Or maybe they do have symptoms, but they don't connect them to the notion of transmittable pathogens. A third possibility lies in their past history: they may have ceased having symptoms of a particular physical illness or complaint long ago, but they become asymptomatic carriers of pathogens relating to that condition. Many of these pathogens are still discharged into sexual secretions.

Once we accept the fact that horizontally transmitted bacteria can cause infertility as well as other major illnesses, it's little wonder that the rate of infertility and the rate of infection-driven illnesses have climbed so dramatically over the past thirty years. That same period—the era of the birth control pill and the sexual liberation movement—has witnessed the sharpest increase in sexual activity in modern times. For example, statistics kept by the Centers for Disease Control and Prevention show that the rate of sexual intercourse during teenage high school years has risen from an estimated 30 percent in 1971 to 46 percent in 2001 (with a spike to 54 percent in 1991, before fear of AIDS and use of condoms became more widespread) [19].

Vertical transmission features a child becoming infected in the contaminated environment of the mother's uterus or birth canal. In the latter case, the actual source of the infection could be either the mother or the father or both, due to the possibility of horizontal transmission of pathogens between them, either prior to, or during, the pregnancy. The child can then carry the infectious agents into his or her adulthood, at which time he or she may begin passing them on to others both horizontally and vertically.

These definitions of horizontal and vertical transmission sound very clinical. But behind the dry language are some astounding implications that we'll examine in detail in later chapters of this book. Among them are the following facts:

- The fetus can be contaminated with vertically transmitted pathogens that cause a variety of major illnesses, including infertility, various kinds of cancers, diabetes and heart disease. This makes the prenatal period even more critical in determining a child's lifetime physical, mental, emotional, and reproductive health than experts previously realized. And it places on prospective parents even greater responsibility to make certain they don't transmit pathogens to each other or their child.

- By charting our own personal health and sexual history and, as best we can, the histories of our partner(s), siblings, parents, and even grandparents, we can determine how likely we are to be carrying such infectious agents.

- Because many of the same agents that trigger serious medical diseases also have the capacity to cause conditions leading to infertility, our history-taking can tell us whether we are at high, medium, or low risk of experiencing—and passing on to our children—not only infertility, but also other major diseases.

- The more diseases we have in our family history, the more likely we are to experience infertility problems.

Even if you have already identified a particular condition as the cause of your infertility—for example, pelvic inflammatory disease or idiopathic low sperm count—it is crucial to investigate the possibility that vertically or horizontally transmitted bacteria may also be a factor. Fortunately this investigation, from both a personal and a medical standpoint, is relatively easy and inexpensive.

Once you complete the questionnaires in Chapter 7 of this book to your best ability, you'll have an excellent tool for beginning to identify possible pathogens. You can then share it with your doctor and other members of your medical team. Ask for antibiotic therapy to reduce or eliminate those pathogens, as it is potentially the most effective and certainly the safest, least invasive, and least expensive treatment associated with regaining fertility. You'll learn more about how it works in Chapter 4.

CAN DIET, EXERCISE, AND LIFESTYLE CHANGES HELP?

Is there anything you can start doing or not doing right now, even before you read the rest of this book, to increase your chances of achieving a pregnancy?

Prospective parents read and hear all sorts of claims about everyday products, activities, practices, or experiences that may assist or hinder their ability to conceive. If only to give you some peace of mind and a properly skeptical perspective on the subject as soon as possible, it makes sense to address the more common claims here in the first chapter, although other pertinent information is given in later sections of the book. These claims are organized below by general topic:

DIET: Excess obesity in men is associated with lower sperm count (fat tissue converts androgen, a male hormone, into estrogen, a female hormone). Anorexia and/or bulimia in women can lead to disruption of the menstrual cycle.

Unless obesity is associated with distinct clinical syndromes, such as hypogonadism or polycystic ovarian disease, no particular foods (including soybeans), dietary patterns, or eating habits have been linked one way or the other to fertility or infertility. There is also no conclusive evidence that caffeine, aspartame, or short-term nutritional deficiencies cause problems.

EXERCISE: In men, only a lack of exercise contributing to obesity (see above) can lead, indirectly, to infertility. In women, only excessive exercise leading to extremely low weight can result in inability to conceive. Aside from these extreme situations, no particular regimen or form of exercise or physical positioning during or after inter-course on either individual's part can improve the odds of achieving a pregnancy. However, regular exercise of any kind can help reduce an individual's stress level, and a high stress level has been shown to have a negative influence on a woman's ovulation, a man's ability to perform sexually, and either partner's interest in sexual intercourse. I'll have more to say about stress in a moment.

ALCOHOL AND RECREATIONAL DRUGS: In men, heavy cocaine use can temporarily depress the sperm count. Heavy marijuana or alcohol use can also reduce sperm production as well as lower the output of testosterone. In men and women, heavy marijuana use can lower the secretion of a pituitary hormone involved in activating reproductive functions.

During a pregnancy, women are advised to abstain from alcohol consumption altogether because of the risk of passing along fetal alcohol syndrome to the child. Cocaine has also been shown to have adverse effects on a pregnancy but not on a woman's ability to conceive.

PRESCRIPTION DRUGS: [Table 1] In men, the commonly used drugs spironolactone, nitrofurantoin, sulfarmethoxazole, tetracycline, and anabolic steroids can adversely impact sperm quality. In addition, beta-blockers, phentolamine, methyldopa, quinidine, and reserpine can interfere with ejaculatory function. On average, it takes three to six months after usage for the effects of these drugs to wear off. In women, the effects of these drugs, if any, on reproductive function-ing is still poorly understood.

	Generic	Brand	Company
Spirinolactone	Spirinolactone		Mylan
	Spirinolactone and Hydrochlorothyazide		Mylan
	Spirinolactone		Geneva
Nitrofurantoin	Nitrofurantoin monohydrate	Macrobid Capsules	P&G Pharmaceuticals
Sulfamethoxazole		Bactrim Pediatric Suspension	Roche
		Bactrim Tablets	Roche
		Bactrim DS	Roche
		Septra Suspension	Monarch
		Septra Grape Suspension	Monarch
		Septra Infusion	Monarch
	Sulfamethoxazole and Trimethoxazole tablets		Watson
	Sulfamethoxazole Injectable		Elkins-Sinn
Tetracycline		Helidac Therapy	Prometheus
	Tetracycline hydrochloride capsules		Mylan
Beta Blockers		Betapace	Berlex
		Blocadren	Merck
		Brevibloc	Baxter
		Corgard	Monarch
		Inderal	Wyeth-Ayerst
		Nadolol	Mylan
		Tenormin	Astra-Zeneca
		Toprol	Astra-Zeneca
		Zebeta	Lederle
Beta blockers with diuretics		Corzide	Monarch
		Timolide	Merck
		Ziac	Lederle
Alpha blocker	Phentolamine	Regitine	Novartis
Methyldopa	Methyldopa		Mylan
	Methyldopa and Hydrochloride		Mylan
		Aldocor	Merck
Quinidine	Quinidine Sulfate		Watson
	Quinidine Gluconate		Watson
Reserpine		Diutensine-R	Wallace

Table 1. Prescription drugs interfering with male fertility.

CIGARETTE SMOKING: In women, heavy ` cigarette smoking impairs the ability to conceive and increases the risk not only of complications during pregnancy, but also of harm to the unborn child. In men, cigarette smoking has no apparent effect on the ability to conceive.

EXPOSURE TO HEAT OR COLD: In men and women, infertility cannot be scientifically associated with the use of hot tubs, saunas, or electric blankets. In addition, the common belief that men can "cook" their sperm by wearing tight-fitting underwear or sitting too long in one position has not been clinically proven. This means that a man doesn't necessarily improve his chances of assisting conception by substituting boxer shorts for bikini briefs, or by putting an ice pack on his driver-seat cushion.

Some men suffering from varicocele have managed to overcome their infertility after wearing an ether-filled cooling device directly applied to the swollen, heat-generating veins for an extended period of time. However, this relatively crude overriding strategy can become problematic when it enables pathogen-laden sperm, previously confined in the testicles, to infect the female partner. The result can be an even more complicated case of secondary infertility, possibly involving a miscarriage or the birth of an unhealthy child.

EXPOSURE TO CHEMICALS AND OTHER ORGANIC COMPOUNDS: In men, excessive exposure to environmental toxins, including pesticides, has been found to have a negative impact on sperm formation, but this is rarely if ever a concern for the average home dweller. There has also been no evidence of male- or female-related infertility due to Agent Orange contamination. In women, neither environmental toxins nor cosmetics (including hair dye, hairspray, and nail polish) have been linked to infertility. Abusive inhalation of solvents during pregnancy can cause toxicity problems for the embryo, but no data associates such abuse with a failure to conceive.

EXPOSURE TO HEAVY METALS: No link has yet been established between exposure to heavy metals (like mercury or lead) and a man's or a woman's infertility. However, if a woman is exposed to heavy metals while pregnant, there is an increased risk of fetal toxicity and malformation, as well as stillbirth or miscarriage.

RADIATION AND CHEMOTHERAPY: Neither men nor women have been shown to suffer infertility-causing side effects from the low radiation doses delivered by standard x-ray or electronic scanning equipment. However, high-dose radiation (like radiation therapy for testicular cancer) can lead to temporary or permanent damage in sperm production. Chemotherapy, which has a strong impact on the entire body, can likewise lead to temporary or permanent infertility in both men and women [20-24].

BLOOD TRANSFUSIONS: Because blood transfusions can introduce infectious bacteria into any and all parts of a person's body, they can indirectly lead to conditions that cause infertility in both men and women.

Two final subjects relating to the prevention of infertility need to be mentioned: **good hygiene** and conservative, **sexually responsible conduct**. Because infectious agents play such a major role in causing infertility, it makes sense that the more we avoid or the better we manage situations that can lead to infections of any kind, the less chance we will have of developing the types of infections that can compromise our reproductive capability. Ideally, beginning in our childhood, we should make sure to keep our bodies and home environment clean, wash our hands often, change our under clothes at least every day, and do what we can to maintain good physical health. Then, assuming we don't remain chaste until marriage to an equally chaste partner, we should keep our number of sexual partners to a minimum and use condoms (the safest form of contraception) during intercourse.

Human nature being what it is, this is advice that may not be easy to hear, much less apply to one's own life. And, regrettably, by the time an individual or couple is dealing with infertility, much infectious damage has probably already been done. Nevertheless, these recommendations remain sound and helpful ones to adopt no matter how late you may feel you are in coming to them.

STRESS MANAGEMENT: GETTING OFF TO A GOOD START

I've already referred to the fact that a high level of stress can compromise an individual's fertility. Whether the source of the negative stress is work pressure, family tension, a personal crisis, or simply the struggle to conceive or bear a child, the result can be complex psychological and physiological reactions that upset the normal course of sexual relations and possibly even reproductive functioning.

For decades this problem has been virtually ignored by fertility specialists. The reason is understandable: modern science has so far been unable to design a survey or experiment that can measure what correlations, if any, exist between stress and infertility.

A similar but not quite as pronounced difficulty applies to more serious psychological problems. Based on the information we have so far, it seems unlikely that such problems can be a significant cause of infertility, although they can be an effect when the individual or couple doesn't accept the situation or deal with it constructively. Certain strong emotions, like severe depression, have shown themselves capable of causing hormonal changes that can result in infertility, but this kind of scenario is very rare.

As for stress, its precise nature is even harder to define than psychological conditions like depression, so its effect on different kinds of minds and bodies is all the more resistant to calculation. Nevertheless, anecdotal evidence and clinical observation have increasingly indicated that a high level of stress experienced by either or both partners may contribute to a couple's infertility. And if it doesn't, it remains a serious problem for the infertile people involved—one that may only grow worse as they continue to live with a diagnosis of infertility and to undergo ever more anxiety-provoking tests, treatments, hardships, and disappointments.

Recently, a growing number of fertility specialists have been addressing these truths in their practices. An article in the New York Times on October 8, 2002 reported that approximately half of the 370 fertility centers approved by the Society for Assisted Reproductive Technology have expanded their psychological services in the past two years by hiring psychologists, starting support groups, and launching stress-reduction programs and workshops.

During this same time period, Resolve, a national infertility support organization, experienced a 60 percent increase in calls from infertility patients seeking help in coping with stress. Commenting on this phenomenon, Stephanie Greco, Resolve's director of communications, said, "Infertility has been in the closet for so long, and it's just beginning to come out. There's been more awareness, so people are beginning to feel it's okay to get help, rather than to feel totally helpless and isolated."

To ensure that you are mentally and emotionally more fit to be fertile, or to cope with infertility and its treatments, you would do well to consider up front what you could do to alleviate excess stress, or prevent it from happening, in your own life. You might try eliminating certain problematic activities from your schedule and replacing them with more relaxing ones. Maybe you would benefit from sharing your worries and troubles more openly with one or two close friends. Perhaps you should incorporate more physical exercise into your routine: take a yoga class or go on a short, easy walk at the start or the end of each day. Or possibly you need to treat yourself more often to a movie, a special meal, or an evening of total relaxation.

Some people already know what works to sustain their sanity, spirits, and energy when they feel mentally or emotionally challenged. If you'd like more guidance on these issues, by all means ask your doctor or people you trust for advice. Contact Resolve or other support groups for suggestions. Above all, prepare yourself to have what you'll certainly need in your ongoing campaign to produce and then raise a healthy child: patience, self-reliance, and equanimity.

In addition, do whatever you can to become more informed about—and therefore, empowered to manage—your particular infertility situation. The book you hold in your hands, and the questionnaires it offers, are here to help you in this single most positive, stress-managing endeavor.

CHAPTER 1 REFERENCES

1. CDS's Reproductive Health Information Source. "1999 Assisted Reproductive Technology Success Rate."
2. CDC's Reproductive Health Information Source. "2000 Assisted Reproductive Technology Success Rate."
3. Tough S.C., Green C.A., Svenson L.W., Belik W. "Effect of in vitro fertilization on low birth weight, preterm delivery and multiple births." *Journal of Pediatrics,* 2000 May; 136(5): 618-22.
4. Schive L.A., Meikle S.F., Ferre C. et al. "Low and very low birth weight in infants conceived with use of assisted reproductive technology." *New England Journal of Medicine,* 2002 March 7; 346: 731-737.
5. Isaksson R., Gissler M., Tiitinen A. "Obstetric outcome among women with unexplained infertility after IVF: a matched case-control study." *Human Reproduction,* 2002; 17(7): 1755-61.
6. Paulson R.J., Boostanfar R., Saadat P., et al. "Pregnancy in the sixth decade of life: obstetric outcomes in women of advanced reproductive age." *Journal of the American Medical Association,* 2002 Nov 13; 288(18): 2320-3.
7. Ludwig M., Dietrich K. "Follow-up of children born after assisted reproductive technologies." *Reproductive Biomedicine Online,* 2002 Nov-Dec; 5(3): 317-22.
8. Hansen M., Kurinczuk J. J., Bower C., Webb S. "The risk of major birth defects after intracytoplasmic sperm injection and in vitro fertilization." *N Eng J Med,* 2002 March 7; 346: 725-730.
9. Kuivurova S., Hartikainen A.L., Gissler M., Hemminki E., Sovio U., Jarvelin M.R. "Neonatal outcome and congenital malformations in children born after in-vitro fertilization." *Hum Reprod,* 2002 May; 17(5): 1133-4.
10. Varma T.R., Patel R.H. "Outcome of pregnancies following investigation and treatment of infertility." *International Journal of Gynecology and Obstetrics,* 1987 Apr; 25(2): 113-20
11. Maman E., Lunenfeld E., Levy A., Vardi H., Potashnik G. "Obstetric outcome of singleton pregnancies conceived by in vitro fertilization and ovulation induction compared with those conceived spontaneously." *Fertility and Sterility,* 1998 Aug; 70(2): 240-5
12. National Center for Health Statistics, Series 23, No 19. "Fertility, Family Planning and Women's Health: New Data from the 1995 National Survey of Family Growth."
13. Clause C. Ph.D. "To Have...or Not to Have," *The American Scholar* (Winter 2002), pp. 71-79.
14. National Center for Health Statistics, Vol 50, No 10. "HHS Report Shows Teen Birth Rate Falls to New Record Low in 2001."

15. Ewald P.W., Cochran G. "Catching on to What's Catching." *Natural History*, February 1999, p.34.
16. Mosher W.D., Pratt W.F. "Fecundity and infertility in the United States: incidence and trends." *Fertil Steril* 56:192.1991.
17. Stephen E.H., Chandra A, "Updated projections of infertility in the United States: 1995-2025." *Fertil Steril* 70:30,1998.
18. York J., Devoe M. "Health Issues in Survivors of Prematurity." *Southern Medical Journal*, 2002; 95(9): 969-976.
19. CDC, MMWR, Sept 27, 2002/51(38); 856-859. "Trends in Sexual Risk Behaviors Among High School students – United States, 1991-2001."
20. Foster W.G. "Do environmental contaminants adversely affect human reproductive physiology?" *Journal of Obstetrics and Gynecology of Canada*, 2003 Jan; 25(1): 33-44
21. Neubert D. "Reproductive toxicology: The science today." *Teratogenesis Carcinogenesis Mutagenesis*, 2002; 22(3): 159-74.
22. Axmon A., Rylander L., Stromberg U., Hagmar L. "Female fertility in relation to the consumption of fish contaminated with persistent organochlorine compounds." *Scandinavian Journal of Work, Environment & Health* 2002; 28(2): 124-32.
23. Petrelli G., Mantovani A. "Environmental risk factors and male fertility and reproduction." *Contraception*, 2002; 165 (4): 297-300.
24. Lindbohm M.L., Sallmen M., Taskinen H. "Effect of exposure to environmental tobacco smoke on reproductive health." *Scand J Work Environ Health*, 2002; 28 Suppl 2: 84-96.

CHAPTER 2

THE HEART OF THE MATTER: VERTICALLY AND HORIZONTALLY TRANSMITTED INFECTIONS

Know thyself.

—*Inscription above the oracle at Delphi*

Each couple's infertility is a puzzle of unique factors that either or both of the partners bring to the situation. In all too many cases, however, each couple's response to a diagnosis of infertility is the same. Understandably frustrated, fearful, and desperate, the would-be parents feel pressured to identify and blame a specific malfunction in the reproductive process and then utilize all scientific means to correct or work around it.

Regrettably, many of their physicians feel a similar urgency. After all, their training prepares them to solve medical dilemmas as expeditiously as possible. They are obligated to take cues from their patients, and their professional reputations as birth facilitators are at stake.

In contrast to this compulsion-driven scenario, however, lies a more sensible and potentially far more beneficial approach to infertility: namely, a fundamental, broad-based, and humane exploration of the mystery itself. Before focusing attention on isolated, end-of-the-line complications like sluggish sperm, poorly developed uterine lining, problems with egg production, the infertile partners and their medical team would do well to pay more attention to the basic, underlying question, "What are all the relevant factors that the individual partners are bringing to the situation?"

The answer is not immediately found in test tubes, culture smears, or sonogram scans. Instead, it starts revealing itself in each partner's personal and family history.

As someone who is concerned about being infertile, you need to start by recalling your own physical illnesses in the past and your own history of sexual partners and child-conceiving efforts. You then need to gather as much similar information as you can pertaining to your siblings, parents, and even grandparents.

What can the resulting data about isolated, repeated, or chronic health problems tell you and your doctor? It can reveal signs that harmful bacteria or other microscopic pathogens have been passed along to you by other people, even your own parents and grandparents. Chances are excellent that these destructive agents are still present in your body, complicating your life, your partner's life, and any new life the two of you attempt to create.

What Damage Can Pathogens Do?

Tracking down evidence of pathogenic infection in your personal and family history is a relatively simple quest, as you'll discover in this book, but it's a very important one, especially for would-be parents. Pathogens are primary or secondary culprits in the vast majority of infertility cases. Any indication of possible or actual transmission that you uncover will help medical specialists determine the answers to several critical questions:

- Are pathogens now, or could they become, a root or contributing cause of reproductive problems you experience?

- Which pathogens are the most likely culprits?

- How, specifically, are they hindering, or could they hinder, your efforts to conceive or to have a successful pregnancy?

- What other health threats might they pose to yourself and any child you produce (as well as, in many cases, any child you have already produced)?

- How are infections from these pathogens best treated?

Simply put, pathogens are tiny organisms—invisible, intangible, and often undetectable—that can live throughout the human body and do a great deal of harm. They come in different categories (like bacteria, viruses, prions, and so on) and, within each category, go by different names (like Chlamydia, Mycoplasma, anaerobic bacteria, and so on). For the most part, however, they are each capable of causing a distinct set of problems in human reproductive systems.

Within women's bodies, these pathogens can easily create hardened, thickened tissues. Medically known as adhesions, they can block or scar the ovaries, in which case they may hinder ovulation, damage the eggs, or harm the fallopian tubes, making it difficult or impossible for eggs to descend from the ovaries and unite with sperm [1, 2].

Pathogenic infections can also trigger a host of other problems leading to female infertility, including:

- Endometriosis: In my opinion, this is the most insidious form of pelvic infection, caused by a variety of bacteria. The affected areas show an abnormal growth of the uterine lining outside the uterus.

- Pelvic Inflammatory Disease (PID): This disease is characterized by the infectious swelling of tissue anywhere in the reproductive system, with subsequent structural destruction and the formation of adhesions (scar tissue). Scar tissue can form inside the uterus. A severe case is referred to as Asherman's syndrome.

- Poor development of the uterine lining: Either ovarian hormone deficiency or a uterine lining that fails to respond causes this clinical condition known as luteal phase defect.

- Poor cervical mucus: The mucus-filled cervix is the gateway between the vagina and the uterus. When infected, the mucus kills, damages, or retards sperm.

- Painful vaginal swelling: This condition can make inter-course impossible.

- Irregularities in hormone production: Among the irregulari-ties are any changes in cycle length; time of ovulation; color, pattern, duration, or pain associated with the menstrual flow; and any development of, or changes in, PMS symp-toms.

- Immunological infertility develops as a secondary phenome-non due to previous infections.

Within men's bodies, the same pathogens can cause significant harm to semen quality, negatively affecting its volume, sperm struc-ture (medically known as morphology), and ability to move (motili-ty). Pathogenic infections can change the viscosity of the ejaculate, which can greatly interfere with the fertilizing capacity of the sperm. They can also damage the testicles and cause adhesions that block or scar the sperm ducts. Infections in the urethra and prostate can make erection and ejaculation painful to the point where intercourse is impossible. [3, 4, 5]

In Chapter 4, I explain how specific pathogens and pathogenic problems are diagnosed and treated. In this chapter, we'll look at the preceding human picture—how bacteria get transmitted from one individual to another, and how, in general, they contribute to infer-tility and other adverse health conditions. It's a picture you'll be developing for yourself and any infertility specialist you consult as you begin thinking about your own personal and family health his-tory, where any number of pathogens may lurk.

HORIZONTAL TRANSMISSION: PARTNER TO PARTNER

The most well known way in which an individual's reproductive system can become infected with pathogens is through sexual con-tact with another person whose reproductive system is already infected. This mode of transmission is called horizontal because it occurs between two "peers" or partners. Unfortunately, the infected person is not often aware that he or she harbors these microscopic troublemakers, nor is there any observable indication to an outsider.

Whatever internal havoc they may be wreaking, externally they yield no symptoms.

The current definition of sexually transmitted diseases (STD) is too narrow to cover all the kinds of pathogens that can cause trouble. This definition includes the well-known villains chlamydia, gonorrhea, and syphilis, all of which can trigger damage within the genital tract and at least one of which is present in over half of the cases of pelvic inflammatory disease [6]. However, there are also sexually transmitted aerobic and anaerobic bacteria that pose an equally significant threat to reproduction. Group B streptococcus, for example, can wreak havoc in the reproductive process, even though it doesn't cause actual structural damage.

Pathogens travel in the body fluids associated with sexual intercourse. Once they've made the journey to a new reproductive system, they can lodge there and spread on their own initiative, sometimes assisted or hindered by other developments or factors in the system (we'll identify some of these possibilities later in the chapter).

Because of the mechanics of male-female intercourse, with the penis penetrating the vagina and directly injecting the seminal fluid, an infection much more readily passes from the man to the woman than the other way around. However, either partner is capable of giving an infection to the other.

What's more, even though repeated sexual contact between the same two partners increases the odds that an infection will be transmitted between them in either direction, one partner can pass along representatives of his or her entire load of pathogens to the other partner in a single sexual act. This fact puts a definite premium on virginity, abstinence, selective sexual activity, and the intelligent use of birth control methods. While individual immune systems differ greatly in their capacity to handle invasive pathogens, it's fair to say in general that the more sexual partners a person has, the more likely he or she is to experience contamination of the genital tract.

At the very least, it's wise to use birth control methods that help prevent infections from being horizontally transmitted. Consistent use of condoms offers the greatest protection, although a small risk continues to exist. Other forms of birth control still allow for the exchange of genital secretions and, therefore, infectious agents. I'll note the particular influence of birth control pills on pathogenic infections in a moment. First, let's consider the different ways that infections take hold and spread after they are introduced into a person's reproductive system. (For anatomical reference see Figures 1, 2 and 3.)

The situation for a man is fairly straightforward. Once the pathogens enter his urethra, they can then easily spread throughout this passageway and cause painful urination, urethral discharge, and discomfort with ejaculation. On the next level the infection can spread to the prostate gland, resulting in acute or chronic prostatitis. The healthy prostate serves as both a mechanical and an immunological barrier that prevents urethral bacteria from reaching and contaminating the internal male sex organs. Highly pathogenic bacteria, however, can cross this barrier and generate such adverse conditions as seminal vesiculitis, epidydimitis, and ultimately even orchitis (inflammation of the testes).

For a woman carrying horizontally or vertically acquired bacteria, the unfolding of possible events is more complicated. The female reproductive system is also divided into two compartments that can be separated from each other. The lower compartment is the vagina. The upper one consists of the uterine cavity, ovaries, and fallopian tubes.

Separating the two compartments is the cervix, an important immunological and mechanical barrier. The mucus filling and covering the vaginal portion of the cervix is highly hostile to sperm, keeping it from reaching the upper compartment throughout the menstrual cycle except when eggs are being released (ovulation) and during menstruation itself. While this sperm-barrier exists, infections can only be transmitted to, or spread within, the lower compartment (unless the bacteria involved are especially pathogenic and fast-growing). When the mucus is favorable to the passage of sperm, the sperm can carry infectious agents into the upper compartment: either pathogens they brought with them from the man, or ones they acquired from the woman's lower genital tract.

A pregnancy also opens up the entire reproductive system, so that pathogens previously confined to the lower compartment, or new infectious agents altogether, can invade the upper compartment. During conception, sperm transfer infectious agents from the lower to the upper compartment. After pregnancies, including one terminated by the earliest possible miscarriage or abortion, both the upper and lower reproductive compartments are exposed to the infection.

The proper use of a diaphragm during sexual activity confines sperm—and any pathogens they carry—to the lower compartment, even during ovulation. Birth control pills, by virtue of sustaining hostile cervical mucus, also keep sperm from traveling into the upper compartment, except when intercourse takes place during menstruation. Typically, however, women using the birth control pill with multiple partners develop an infected cervix, a condition that comes to haunt them later when they attempt to conceive a child.

Special circumstances also affect the spread of pathogens from one compartment to another. A woman who suffers from a chronic cervical infection, keeping the mucus hostile to sperm, is relatively safe from upper compartment infection during unprotected intercourse. The same infection will also serve as a form of birth control.

However, if this woman receives antibiotic therapy, either for the cervical infection or an unrelated condition, there is a chance that the cervical mucus will recover enough to allow sperm to pass through the cervix. If that opening occurs before the cervical infection or any other lower compartment infection is completely eradicated, the previously safe and sheltered upper tract will swiftly become contaminated, resulting in possible damage to the endometrium, ovaries, and fallopian tubes.

Another way in which infections can bypass the cervix is through the application of assisted reproductive technology, most commonly intrauterine insemination. In the latter procedure, sperm are injected directly into the upper compartment precisely to override a hostile cervical environment. The sad result, with or without a subsequent pregnancy, is the transmission of pathogens into the upper compartment by means of the injected sperm. In file after file of my female patients who came to me after having intrauterine insemination elsewhere, I see that the insemination was rapidly followed by deterioration of the uterine lining function, development of tubal damage, and/or ovarian hormone irregularities.

In the world of infertility treatment, nothing bothers me more than the fact that so many of my colleagues ignore or fail to respect the critical role that the cervical environment plays in blocking or regulating the spread of infectious agents. I regard the cervix as a uniquely significant part of a woman's reproductive system, not only in governing the migration of sperm to the egg in order to achieve pregnancy, but also in protecting the upper compartment from an advancing infection.

I'm also impressed with the manner in which the cervix can indirectly protect a contaminated upper compartment from further deterioration. I've witnessed a number of cases in which an infection-fueled dysfunction in the upper compartment advanced to the point where the cervix finally shut down due to this infection. From then on, the functioning stabilized, thanks to the cervix preventing any further infection by newly arriving sperm.

Here's how this kind of case progresses: at the beginning of a couple's trial for a pregnancy, a test of the woman's cervical mucus soon after intercourse (called a "post-coital test") shows that it is normal. As months pass without a pregnancy occurring, the woman reports drastic changes in all aspects of her menstrual period: color, pattern, interval, pain, and associated PMS symptoms. These changes peak around the time that another post-coital test turns poor, due to the development of chronic cervicitis. From then on there is no further worsening of symptoms, unless artificial insemination is administered to bypass the hostile mucus.

The remaining infection in both compartments of the woman's reproductive system can then be cured by a sufficient course of antibiotics. The key word is "sufficient." An incomplete, too-short course may only partially clear up the cervical infection to the point where bacteria-laden sperm can pass through to the upper compartment, which in turn becomes more contaminated than it was before treatment. Thus the woman's symptoms will start to worsen again.

A couple of other special circumstances relating to horizontal transmission are also worth noting. One is called "the boomerang effect." Through urination and ejaculation, a man's comparatively simple genital tract is rinsed free of a certain percentage of its bacterial load on a regular basis. In a woman's more compartmentalized system, the vaginal pool, with the cervix as its stopper, serves as a constant brewing medium where bacteria multiply and fester.

Let's assume "Alan" transmits pathogenic bacteria to "Alice," and her cervix and vagina get infected. Eventually Alice's vaginal pool develops a much higher colony count of Alan's bacteria than he has himself at any one time. Alice transmits these bacteria back to Alan. Soon he develops his first ever genital tract infection. Why? Because he now hosts a much greater number of bacteria than can be held in check by the combination of routine rinsing and the normal functioning of his own immune system. In summary, Alan has been "boomeranged" by his own bacteria. Pregnancy puts a woman into an immune-suppressed state, which allows vaginal bacteria to proliferate, sometimes leading to unexplained urethritis, prostatitis or epididymitis in the male partner, if the couple remains sexually active during the pregnancy.

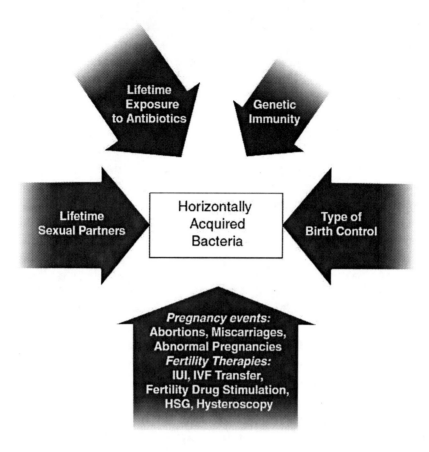

Figure 1 — Factors determining the horizontally acquired bacterium flora.

The other special circumstance involves the sperm count. Because sperm can carry pathogens into and through the female reproductive system, it makes sense that a higher number of sperm translates into a greater chance for transmission. A man who has no sperm in his seminal fluid (azoospermia) can only contaminate a female genital tract up to the cervical level, because the pathogen-laden fluid itself doesn't travel any further. By contrast, a man with a high sperm count can trigger a very rapid deterioration of the female genital tract above the cervix. Somewhere in between is the situation of a man with a low sperm count (oligospermia). For summary of factors affecting horizontal transmission see Figure 1.

Laura and Eli: A Case of Horizontal Transmission

One particular case involving a couple that came to my office represents well what damage can happen when an impeccably fertile female reproductive canal is exposed to infected seminal fluid. In fact, it shows the whole gamut of changes that a female pelvic area can exhibit during a gradually progressing bacterial infection. If the woman involved had been more aware that this kind of pattern could occur—as aware as you will be after reading this book—she could have self-diagnosed her problem very early in the process and sought the proper help to keep it from getting worse.

Laura was brought up in a strict Roman Catholic family and absorbed its moral code of no premarital sex and absolute sexual fidelity to one's spouse. By the time she consulted me, her two older brothers and her younger sister, all married, had each produced more than one healthy child: a sign that the family line was almost certainly free of the kind of vertically transmitted pathogens that can lead to infertility.

Shortly after her twentieth birthday, Laura wed her high school sweetheart, Tom. They had two healthy children together before the marriage ended in divorce. A couple of years later Laura married Eli, the second sexual partner in her life. Her reproductive health started noticeably deteriorating even during the honeymoon, when she developed an annoying vaginal infection.

At the time, Laura had just begun using a birth control pill, and she blamed it for the infectious symptoms she was feeling. For a while she got relief by applying creams to the irritated surface. Later, when the creams no longer worked, she simply learned to live with the problem. She was eventually diagnosed with cystitis (cause unknown), which she treated with one daily tablet of Macrodantin (a so-called maintenance therapy).

Laura's symptoms abated and, because she and Eli were not yet ready to have a child, she kept using the birth control pill. Over the next four years, she continued to have minor cystitis symptoms from time to time. She also had one major scare: a pap test showed pre-cancerous changes. A colposcopy examination and subsequent cone biopsy, however, revealed nothing more then a severe local inflammation.

When Laura turned 37, she and Eli decided to have a child, feeling it was now or never because of her age, so she stopped taking the birth control pill and the couple began trying to conceive. After six months with no success, they consulted a colleague of mine, who referred them to me for a post-coital test.

I gave the couple my usual instructions relating to post-coital testing: monitor ovulation with a predictor kit, have intercourse the night after the colors turns red, and come to the office the next morning. I spotted trouble in the first test: there were no sperm in a mostly cloudy cervical mucus that was loaded with white blood cells. Forced to question whether intercourse had taken place at all, I used donor sperm to test the mucus. The stickiness of that mucus prevented even the best donor sperm from penetrating it, despite the fact that it was the correct time for ovulation.

I immediately explored the possibility of an infection. Cultures showed that the mucus was saturated with pathogenic bacteria, mostly anaerobic, identical to those recovered from Eli's seminal fluid. So I prescribed an oral antibiotic regimen. A month later, I saw slightly better results in another post-coital test: A few sperm were penetrating a still obviously infected cervical mucus.

Before the menstruation even occurred, however, a new kind of trouble appeared. Laura called my office to say that her period was four days late but repeated urine tests were negative for pregnancy. In addition, she complained of a bloated and full lower abdomen. When her period finally started a few days later, it began with two days of staining and then the usual four days of heavy flow. The end of the period was again four days of staining.

I didn't see Laura again for four months, during which time she continued to work with my colleague. He had advised her to override the problematic cervical mucus by means of artificial insemination. Laura had therefore been regularly taking Clomid and receiving at least two inseminations per month.

Sadly, the result was not a conception but a dramatic worsening of Laura's reproductive health. She had never before had premenstrual syndrome (PMS), but now she experienced one of its classic symptoms: a long (in her case, 14 days) period of nervous irritability prior to her menstruation. Also, in the week preceding her period, her breasts hurt and she gained at least five pounds of weight, mostly water. The menstruation in itself had changed drastically. The flow was now diminished to a staining of three days.

To make matters worse, Laura had lost her sexual desire and was almost incapable of lubricating prior to intercourse. The final blow, the one that had led her to contact me again, came when she began losing her hair.

Since Laura's visit coincided with ovulation, I looked at her cervical mucus again. It barely existed, and what little I could recover was sticky and void of sperm and even a donor sperm couldn't penetrate it. A sonogram showed huge, persisting ovarian cysts on both sides and an inactive uterine lining much thinner than it should have been at this "high" time in her cycle. Later, culture studies of the mucus showed an even denser profusion of anaerobic bacteria.

From what I knew so far about Laura's reproductive history, I could mentally reconstruct what had happened to her. The original infection came from Eli's seminal fluid while Laura was on the birth control pill. The bacteria in that fluid rendered her cervical mucus hostile to sperm penetration. The problem was slightly alleviated by the antibiotic treatment I'd prescribed, but that treatment wasn't extensive enough to prevent the infection from reasserting itself. Later, Laura's repeated artificial inseminations brought large amounts of infected seminal fluid directly into the upper genital tract, which had previously been protected by the hostile cervical mucus. The inevitable, disastrous consequences were all the new and more serious upper compartment symptoms Laura was experiencing, signaling the complete and irreversible loss of fertility.

Meagan and Clark: Horizontal Transmission and Secondary Infertility

The case of Laura and Eli illustrates how a horizontally transmitted pathogen can prevent a couple from conceiving any children from the beginning of their relationship. The following case deals with how a horizontally transmitted infection can create secondary infertility, a more subtle, often overlooked condition in which a couple becomes unable to conceive—or give birth to—a baby after having already produced one or more children.

Meagan was sexually active during her college years. One time she experienced a slight vaginal irritation and went to the college clinic, where she was given a routine, seven-day course of the antibiotic doxycycline. The trouble disappeared.

At age 28, Meagan married Clark. Within a few months she was pregnant and, after a seemingly uncomplicated pregnancy, her daughter Gail was born. No one paid much attention to the fact that the birth occurred two weeks early and required an emergency cesarean section: although Meagan had a large pelvis, her cervix didn't dilate beyond two centimeters, even following 18 hours of pitocin stimulation.

The post-operative pain of the cesarean section was obliterated by the joy of parenting a newborn. It is my belief that one of nature's ingenious family-planning strategies is to make young children angelically beautiful by their second birthday. This period allows for the optimum recovery of the female reproductive canal with less bother to the new mother and, therefore, a greater chance that she'll want to have another child.

Sure enough, Meagan was again pregnant just after Gail's second birthday. All went well until the middle of the third month, when the baby's heart stopped beating. No cause could be established, but a second sonogram a few days later confirmed a case of fetal demise. Her gynecologist quickly recommended a D&C. He also assured Meagan and Clark that such events happened all the time without signifying anything negative about future fertility. He advised them to try for another baby as soon as possible.

A good patient, Meagan followed the advice with no success. The case presented an unsolvable puzzle to all the experts she consulted. While doctor after doctor pored over her case history, her reproductive health gradually began to unravel.

No longer did Meagan experience periods with her usual clockwork regularity. Her menstrual bleeding, which used to occur without any preceding symptoms, became an absolving relief to a host of bothersome premenstrual complaints. Her stomach started bloating immediately after ovulation and stayed bloated until the following period. During those same days, her bras did not fit her swollen and extremely tender breasts.

Soon Meagan's periods devolved from five days of bleeding to two days of staining. The only positive change—at least in terms of the pain she felt—was that she no longer had cramps. Instead, she developed mood swings severe enough to send her to a psychiatrist, who called them "natural reactions to reproductive failure."

By this time, Meagan's sexual drive was completely gone. She had barely enough emotional reserve left to care for Gail. It took all Meagan's self-control to keep her PMS reactions at bay while she was around her daughter. Six months prior to consulting me, she and Clark had begun seeing a marriage counselor to prevent a divorce that, nevertheless, appeared more and more inevitable.

During my initial consultation with Meagan and Clark, the history-taking alone convinced me that the series of problems Meagan had suffered—all the way back to the vaginal itching she'd had in college—could be traced to the horizontal transmission of an infection. Both Meagan and Clark were products of normal, full-term pregnancies occurring within highly fertile families, which argued against the possibility of vertical transmission. Cultures of Meagan's body fluids revealed high numbers of Chlamydia bacteria—one of the most virulent pathogens—and here's the chain of events that I reconstructed after that discovery:

Meagan acquires chlamydia from one of her sexual partners during college. It causes only mild discomfort. Because she is using birth control pills, it doesn't spread to her upper genital tract. She receives inadequate treatment for the infection: only the symptoms go away. The infection itself, however, does not; and since there's no follow-up culture at the clinic, this fact goes undetected. She becomes a carrier for chlamydia in the lower genital tract.

Meagan and Clark marry. Clark fails to acquire Meagan's infection. Meagan's upper tract remains pathogen-free and, according to plan, she quickly becomes pregnant. The fertilizing sperm, however, carry bacteria into the uterine cavity. The fetus (Gail) implants in a virtually clean uterus, but as the pregnancy advances, both the fetal cells and the bacteria multiply rapidly, thanks to the natural suppression of Meagan's immune system.

Signs of uterine contamination are overlooked at the time of Gail's delivery: the presence of bacteria affects the time of delivery and profoundly interferes with uterine contractions.

Because Gail is delivered by cesarean section, she escapes being infected while passing through Meagan's vagina. She therefore exhibits good health.

Following the delivery, Meagan's uterine cavity remains filled with bacteria. The count jumps much higher as a result of the second unsuccessful pregnancy as well as other possible very early pregnancies that are quickly lost, during the time span when Meagan and Clark are trying to conceive their second child.

A biopsy of Meagan's uterus confirmed a heavy chlamydia contamination. To combat it, I prescribed an antibiotic regimen (Clindamycin) administered intravenously. I also administered an intrauterine washing using two other antibiotics (Ampicillin and Gentamicin). A ten-day course of an oral antibiotic (Zithromax) completed the therapy.

Afterwards, Meagan reported a complete reversal of her PMS symptoms and normalization of her menstrual flow. Two months later, she became pregnant. On the proper delivery date, a son, Ian, was born vaginally after eight hours of spontaneous labor. He weighed a robust eight pounds and ten ounces at birth, and neither he nor his mother experienced any medical problems in the months to come.

Vertical Transmission: Parent to Child

The other way that infertility-causing pathogens are spread is vertically, from parent to child. Until recently, this route has been under-appreciated and under-investigated. Thanks to a wave of new discoveries, however, that state of affairs is rapidly changing [7-11].

The actual transmission occurs in the mother's reproductive system during pregnancy or delivery, when the child can easily absorb all sorts of infectious agents. The source of these troublemakers, however, can be either the mother or the father, since sexual contact between them enables the father's pathogenic load to infiltrate the mother (horizontal transmission). (For a summary of factors affecting vertical transmission, see Figure 2.)

In fact, given the way vertical transmission works, the true origin of these agents may go back for generations in either or both of the parents' family lines. The result is a chain of intermittent fertility problems that gets passed along until, eventually, there may come a "final generation" individual or couple that can't produce a child.

The way in which a baby is born into the world—the mode of delivery itself—can significantly affect the extent to which pathogens are vertically transmitted. While the fetus is in the uterus, the membranes surrounding it protect it from many pathogens (but not all of them). These membranes naturally rupture during a vaginal delivery, thereby exposing the child as well as the mother's entire reproductive system to a far greater number of pathogens [12].

However, a baby can acquire infections all through the course of the pregnancy. The severity and symptoms of such infections vary greatly depending on the state of his or her immune system at the time of acquisition. If prenatal infants pick up bacteria before they develop an immune system, they become asymptomatic carriers. If they pick up bacteria around the time of their birth, when the immune system is fully functioning, they experience symptomatic

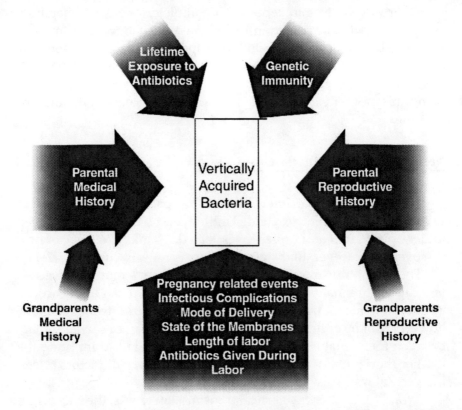

Figure 2—Factors determining the inherited bacterium flora. Note the significance of ancestral bacteria, and medical and reproductive history. The labor process and mode of delivery also plays a critical role.

infections. From my point of view as a doctor, it is sobering to see bodies of Chlamydia bacteria in close proximity to a follicle within an ovarian biopsy specimen. Before an egg can even mature and be fertilized, a villain lurks in its vicinity, poised to strike sooner or later.

When an infection complicates the birth process, interfering with the uterus's natural contractions, the delivery date is likely to come earlier or later than normal. In either case, the length of labor and strength of labor contractions can be influenced considerably after a stimulant like Pitocin is administered. If the membranes rupture early during a lengthy labor, pathogens have all the more time to infect the child prior to his or her delivery. By contrast, rapid deliveries with the membranes rupturing late during labor tend to result in much less seriously-infected newborns.

Babies who are born through cesarean section prior to the rupture of the membranes are spared from a considerable amount of contamination. Records show that they suffer much less from ear infections, tonsillitis, chronic upper respiratory tract problems, colic, or infectious trouble in their urogenital system.

Contrary to popular opinion, most cesarean sections are necessary because an infected uterus is not functioning properly, not because the size of the baby is bigger than the mother's pelvis. This kind of delivery does, however, have the advantage of shielding the baby from even more contamination as well as protecting the mothers' pelvis-supporting muscles from undue wear associated with abnormal labor and delivery.

Because entrenched infections usually create the need for a cesarean section, it makes sense that if a mother has delivered one baby this way, then her subsequent children are also better delivered through caesarean sections, so that they will be less exposed to the pathogens still living in her reproductive system. Given this situation, one could claim that a caesarean-section delivery is a good precaution in any infected pregnancy. The practice is rapidly gaining ground, for example, in the case of HIV-infected pregnancies [13].

Even if such an argument now seems a bit extreme, we can at least appreciate the health advantages of a cesarean-section birth in a pregnancy featuring a widespread infection that causes dysfunctional labor. Once a woman has gone through this type of experience, she doesn't need to repeat it with her next pregnancy as long as she and her partner receive thorough, broad-spectrum antibiotic therapy before the next conception.

In my own practice, I take yet another approach to help reduce the birthing mother's chance of transmitting a series of pathogens. When pregnancy occurs prior to eliminating suspected pathogens from her birth canal, I prescribe appropriate oral or intravenous antibiotics any time during the course of the pregnancy to prevent complications. I also offer repeat cervical cultures at the end of the first and second trimesters. The findings from these cultures can guide the obstetrician to administer the best possible antibiotics during labor and delivery. Ideally, the mother should start receiving them just prior to the rupture of the membranes to prevent any infection from being transmitted to the newborn.

The result of this therapy for the past twenty years has been impressive. Records consistently show fewer complications with pregnancies and little or no transmission of infections from mother to baby. Lately, similar treatment guidelines have been introduced for obstetricians who are dealing with group B streptococcus infections [14].

Now an even more mind-boggling aspect of vertical transmission is beginning to be charted and authenticated. For a long time, clinical records have shown an association between clustered medical problems in a patient's family and a patient's own reproductive problems. As science inches closer to proving that pathogens cause major medical illnesses like heart disease, cancer and diabetes, it becomes more logically apparent that these same pathogens can also cause reproductive problems. Looking at the connection from the opposite angle, we are starting to see that pathogens transmitted vertically can cause, or contribute to, not only infertility, but also other major medical illnesses.

The implications of this new knowledge are astounding. Previously we thought that certain adverse health conditions and reproductive deficiencies were related to genetic, lifestyle, or environmental factors. Now we're discovering that the real troublemakers are very likely infections passed along from mother to child, possibly for generations.

The bottom-line implications for each of us are clear. For one thing, we can find indicators of our possible infertility as well as our possible susceptibility to other illnesses by examining the reproductive and health history of our parents, grandparents, and siblings. For another, we can't consider infertility in isolation from other health problems. As the research articles cited in this book reveal, science is now in the process of proving that pathogens cause or contribute to a wide range of medical illnesses. My own research and clinical observations show that these same infectious agents also cause infertility. If you find, for example, that there's a history of heart disease in your family, it could signal your own predisposition not only to heart disease but also to infertility.

The revolution that has occurred over the past twenty-five years in connecting health problems to pathogens has coincided with my career as a pathologist and infertility specialist, and I have taken an active and even leading part in exploring and verifying this link in my own research and practice. As a means of helping you to understand the nature of vertical transmission and its possible ramifications on a personal level, let me trace how I came to discover more about it and to apply that knowledge effectively in diagnosis and treatment.

By the early 1980s, I had set up a comprehensive microbiology laboratory where I could test biological specimens for all known pathogenic bacteria. I had also developed a very thorough format and style for consulting with patients, including careful and extensive history-taking mechanisms. Nevertheless, one recurring kind of case puzzled me: How could a man whose virginal state at the time of marriage was beyond question seemingly cause a devastating infection in the genital tract of a similarly virginal woman within three months of marriage?

There was no way of explaining this situation without entertaining the possibility of mother-to-daughter or mother-to-son transmission of pathogens within the uterine cavity during the course of the pregnancy or the birthing process. This transmission could have turned the infant into an asymptomatic carrier—one whose developing immune system became tolerant of the pathogenic bacteria involved.

With this in mind, I redesigned my consultative history taking. I introduced new questions about possible pregnancy or labor problems experienced by the mother of each partner. I was looking for signs in the course of pregnancy, labor, or delivery pointing to pathogens in the mother that might have interfered with the process and had a chance to infect the child. Specifically, the new questions focused on the circumstances of conception; the possible prior history of infertility, miscarriages, or ectopic pregnancies; the course of pregnancy itself; and the birth process (for example, whether it featured premature labor, untimely delivery, dysfunctional labor with cesarean section, and/or accompanying infections for either mother or child). A separate part of my redesigned questionnaire dealt with infections affecting other body cavities in early infancy, such as chronic ear infections, tonsillitis, or bronchitis.

Although science had already established that babies could acquire chlamydia, gonorrhea, syphilis, group B streptococcus, and certain other pathogens from the mother's birth canal during the labor process, it was a commonly held belief that unless these pathogens caused symptomatic infections at an early age, later genital tract infection was not possible. A 13-year-old girl named Rachel Leonard was the first of my patients to prove this belief wrong, thanks to the cooperation of her mother.

Rachel, the product of a premature delivery at 37 weeks, had just begun menstruating a few months prior to visiting my office. Her mother sought my help because Rachel suffered persistent vaginal discharge and unbearable cramps with her periods. One morning, I received permission to take specimen swabs from both of their vaginas. Laboratory examination of these swabs proved that mother and daughter had the exact same constellation of pathogens (anaerobic bacteria) in their vaginal fluid.

Here was certain evidence that the mother had transmitted infectious agents to her daughter before her daughter was born, and that they had remained there, undetected and asymptomatic, until over a decade later, when hormonal changes associated with puberty made the environment of Rachel's reproductive system favorable for bacterial growth. The variety and colony count of the anaerobic bacteria identified in both mother and daughter readily justified a diagnosis of bacterial vaginosis and retrospectively explained Rachel's untimely delivery.

Six weeks of antibiotic therapy cleared up Rachel's menstrual problems as well as ovarian cysts that had shown up through sonographic examination. Her mother also opted for the same period of antibiotic therapy, which cleared up her less obvious infection. The ensuing years brought many more virginal girls or young women with genital tract infections to my office. They also had mothers who were willing to go through the testing procedures, and I was able to identify more and more different kinds of pathogens, including Trichomonads, that are capable of being transmitted vertically. I now firmly believe that all pathogens contaminating a mother's uterine cavity can gain access to any of her baby's body cavities, including the reproductive canal.

From the early 1980s onward it was easy for me to trace the negative changes that take place in a woman's reproductive system after it is contaminated by pathogens. Every part of the lower and upper tracts presents a certain set of symptoms, whether the infectious agents were originally acquired vertically or horizontally. One condition, however, was—and in greater part remains—much more difficult to decipher: congenitally depleted ovaries, such as the ones seen in women with primary anovulation, polycystic ovarian syndrome, or any of the subcategories of oligo-anovulatory ovaries. Infertility specialists have had the same difficulty accounting for how men develop congenitally depleted testes, leading to sub-normal semen quality or a suppressed sperm count.

A breakthrough in the latter mystery came for me when an Orthodox Jewish couple, Samuel Schuler, age 19, and his new bride,

Deborah, age 18, consulted me. Both were virgins at the time of their marriage.

Samuel had a very low sperm count and an unusually heavy volume of pathogens growing out of his seminal fluid. Under the microscope, these pathogens also seemed to be attached to his sperm. Typically such problems are attributed to a high degree of sexual experience and episodes of prostate, epididymal, or testicular infections. In his case, those factors clearly didn't apply.

I found the key to Samuel's reproductive health problem in his family history. He was an only child who lost his father, then age 36, to a massive heart attack. His father was also an only child. Samuel's mother had three sisters and a brother, all with impeccable reproductive health histories: each had a large family and no incidence of pregnancy-related problems. His mother, however, presented a different picture altogether. She delivered her first child stillborn at six and a half months and subsequently went through three miscarriages before becoming pregnant with Samuel. He was held in her uterus by means of a cervical stitch, bed rest, and medications for seven and a half months, at which point he was delivered prematurely, a mere five-pounder. Following that, she experienced two more miscarriages.

From this history, I speculated that the reproductive health problems of Samuel's mother as well as Samuel's own low sperm count most likely stemmed from the father. The mother, who came from a highly fertile family and was virginal at the time she married her husband, later exhibited all the cardinal reproductive complications typical of an infected reproductive canal. Since Samuel's father was also virginal at the time of the marriage, the only plausible source for the troublesome pathogens was the father's apparently vertically acquired bacteria. He transmitted these bacteria horizontally to his wife, and she, in turn, transmitted them vertically to their son, Samuel.

But there's an even more fascinating dimension to this case. Knowing how often and how subtly an individual's health problems can be interrelated, I couldn't help thinking that the father's heart attack was somehow connected to his genital tract infection—in other words, that pathogens permeating his body fluids had initiated both problems.

At last I made a significant discovery that helped confirm this connection. First, however, let me give you some background information that will help you appreciate the nature of that discovery. Up until the mid-1970s, it was a routine medical practice to do testicular biopsies on all males who were diagnosed with low sperm count or azoospermia. Before the advent of IVF, a testicular biopsy was the final diagnostic test an infertile couple undertook before being advised to file for adoption. After IVF refinements in the mid-1970s, routine biopsies on testes were largely abandoned. Dr. MacLeod, my predecessor at the clinic I now head, studied hundreds of testicular biopsies during his many decades of active work in male infertility, and he meticulously filed all the semen slides and biopsy tissue blocks he reviewed.

I consulted these files in my multi-stage effort to examine the possibility that the same pathogens could cause a major medical illness like heart disease as well as a reproductive problem. First, I needed to establish that certain kinds of pathogens caused reproductive problems. I began by matching individual semen slides with individual biopsy slides (both slides from the same man). In each case, I then located the paraffin blocks containing the tissues from which these slides were made. I requested new slides to be cut from these tissues and specially stained for bacteria identification: something that wasn't done at the time the previous slides were made. When I looked at these new slides under the microscope, I found what I'd suspected: the particles that showed up on the semen slide were morphologically identical to the particles present in huge numbers on the biopsy slide. I also reviewed my own ovarian biopsy specimens obtained during laparoscopies and had parts of these specimens re-examined with special stains for bacteria. Sure enough, some of these specimens showed the same kinds of bacteria-like particles. In fact, in a high number of infertility patients with ovarian dysfunction, bacteria-like structures were identified in the ovarian biopsy. Through routine cultures of these ovarian biopsy specimens we could identify mycoplasma, Chlamydia and a variety of anaerobic bacteria. This was my first proof that infections caused ovarian trouble.

Next I asked a colleague in the pathology department to secure me a tissue sample of an aorta bearing the kind of plaque associated with heart attacks. The slides were specially stained with Giemsa and Gram technique for bacterial visualization. If my theory were correct, this tissue would contain the same kind of suspected particles that commonly show up in contaminated sperm as well as in testicular and ovarian biopsy specimens. I still recall my excitement as I looked at those stained slides of aortic tissue and saw that the morphology of particles observed there did, indeed, match the morphology of bacteria present in the other slides.

Altogether, these investigations gave me my first, strong lead that medical diseases long assumed to be genetically inherited, like heart disease, might be triggered by pathogens that can be carried through body fluids and, therefore, transmitted to others, including the fetus during pregnancy. My theory, as it evolved from hypothesis to clinical observation and, finally, microscopic documentation, was—and still is—continuously supported by the histories of my patients. One of the major advantages of my lengthy medical practice in the same location is that I've been able to observe several generations in the same family line and, therefore, track all the more closely various interrelated illness patterns and reproductive performance.

Combining my own clinical experience with that of other doctors and with recent scientific discoveries, I am now convinced that the existence of certain maladies and symptoms in an individual's personal or family history may be signs that pathogens are at work in that person's body. These troublemakers are not only the likely source of his or her infertility-related complaints, but also the actual or potential catalysts for other health problems as well.

Analyzing scores of infertility situations and the predictably associated medical diseases, heart disease, high blood pressure, and stroke were the first illnesses that I could put on this list. Later, I was able to add diabetes, pulmonary hypertension, and a host of cancers, such as breast, cervical, uterine, and certain forms of lymphoma. Other illnesses potentially influencing reproductive outcome are chronic cholecystitis, kidney disease and stones, and, on an immunological basis, most of the autoimmune diseases, asthma, and thyroid conditions. Finally, I am convinced that a vertically acquired infection explains the two major puzzles in infertility: low or no sperm count in men (idiopathic oligo/azospermia) and low or no egg production in women (different varieties of oligo/anovulatory ovaries, including the so-called polycystic ovarian syndrome).

I'll discuss these pathogen-related illnesses more thoroughly in the rest of the book, including Chapter 7, which assists you to answer your own medical questionnaires. Let's close this chapter by looking at an example from my files of how vertical transmission works in real life.

Mark and Janine: A Classic Case of Vertical Transmission

Several years ago I was the second fertility specialist consulted by Mark and Janine. They were both physically healthy individuals in their mid-thirties who had not been diagnosed with any medical condition that would account for their infertility. Their previous physician, labeling the cause of their infertility as unknown, had recommended in vitro fertilization. They wanted to pursue my more natural, less risky, and less costly approach.

Exploring Mark's family background, I learned that he is the younger of two siblings, and that his mother suffered one miscarriage just before his birth and another just after. I assumed infection caused the miscarriages, and I knew from past experience that an offspring sandwiched between two miscarriages has a very high chance of acquiring the same infectious agents from the uterine environment.

Continued questioning of Mark revealed that his mother later sought treatment for a chronic gall bladder infection, a frequent late sequel of certain types of pelvic infections caused by bacteria spreading from the genital organs to the inner abdominal structures. When I heard about his mother's menopause, it added another piece of evidence to the puzzle—evidence that the overall problem was infectious contamination. His mother encountered menopause very early (six years before her own mother's onset), and she exhibited unusually severe emotional symptoms as a result. Mark described it as "kind of a nervous breakdown." I've heard countless similar stories regarding that difficult time when a woman's last egg leaves her chronically infected ovaries much sooner then expected and, understandably, she finds it difficult to cope with the sudden hormonal void.

Other indicators of an infectious history emerged in the story of Mark's older sister, who also suffered problems relating to childbearing. Her only son was born six weeks prematurely and turned out to be a sickly child. Later, two early-stage miscarriages ushered in a secondary infertility condition that she was still trying to overcome after four years. I knew a vertically-acquired infection could easily explain her reproductive health problems—the same infection that could be troubling Mark.

Janine's background also betrayed signs of vertically transmitted infection. Her maternal grandparents, who produced six, long-lived children, had no major health or fertility problems. It was a different scenario with her paternal grandparents. On that side, her grand-mother, whose sole child was Janine's father, died of heart disease at the early age of 55. As an adult, Janine's father had chronic prostate infections and, eventually, prostate cancer. Her mother, after giving birth to two children, experienced recurring, abnormally heavy uter-ine bleeding, a medical condition called menometrorrhagia. Repeated surgical procedures failed to correct the bleeding and, to avoid further worsening of an anemic condition, she finally under-went a hysterectomy.

In Janine's history, the route of generation-to-generation infec-tion was almost palpable. As far as Janine could trace it, the major load of bacterial infection apparently spread from her paternal grandmother to her father, who passed it along—via seminal fluid—to her mother, who then transmitted it to Janine. Presumably Janine's one sibling, her 25-year-old sister Mandy, also had it. Although Mandy had not yet tried to have a child, she'd battled severe men-strual cramps and vaginal infections since puberty.

If either Mark's or Janine's family history had been the only one to display evidence of a vertical transmission of infection, it would have offered enough information to explain their current infertility problem. The fact that such evidence manifested itself in both histo-ries made it virtually certain that their difficulty was caused by infec-tious agents.

Tapping my professional knowledge of which infectious agents tend to trigger which illness patterns, I was also better able to deter-mine from Mark's and Janine's histories which particular laboratory tests were most apt to pinpoint the specific troublemakers—in their case, Chlamydia trachomatis and anaerobic bacteria. In addition, I could better gauge what particular intensity and regimen of treat-ment were likely to be the most effective.

The ideal combination of two antibiotics—clindamycin and gen-tamicin—promised to counteract all the offending microorganisms in their systems. After two weeks of intravenous therapy, both Mark's and Janine's follow-up cultures tested negative for pathogen-ic bacteria. Since all infection is accompanied by an immune response—the production of antibodies that are potentially prob-lematic during a conception or pregnancy—it was now up to the state of Mark's and Janine's immune systems to determine when pregnancy could occur. Fortunately, neither of them exhibited signif-icant levels of antibodies. This news meant that they were better prepared to conceive than they had been ever before. Nine months later, I delivered their healthy son.

The key element leading to this successful outcome for Mark and Janine was taking more pains to identify the probable source of their infertility. Specifically, we had to dig more deeply into their personal and family health histories than most doctors normally do. What more powerful argument in favor of history taking can there be?

CHAPTER 2 REFERENCES

1. Cates W. Jr., Rolfs R.T. Jr., Aral S.O. "Sexually Transmitted Diseases, pelvic inflammatory disease, and infertility: an epidemiological update." *Epidemiologic Reviews,* 1990; 12: 199-220.
2. Wasserheit J.N. "Pelvic inflammatory disease and infertility." *Maryland Medical Journal,* 1987; 36: 58-63.
3. Krieger J.N., Ross S.O., Riley D.E. "Chronic prostatitis: epidemiology and role of infection." *Urology,* 2002; 60 (6 Suppl): 8-12.
4. Karkovshy M.E., Pontari M.A. "Theories of prostatitis etiology." *Current Urology Reports,* 2002; 3(4): 307-12.
5. Shafik A. "Demographic and clinical characteristics of men with chronic prostatitis: the National Institute of Health Chronic Prostatitis Cohort study." *Journal of Urology,* 2002; 168(2): 593-8.
6. McCormack W.M. "Pelvic Inflammatory Disease." *New Eng J Med,* 1994; 330: 115-119.
7. Packham C., Gibb D. "Current Concepts: Mother-to-Child Transmission of the Human Immunodeficiency Virus." *N Eng J Med,* 1995; 333: 298-303.
8. Ohto H., Terazawa S., Sasaki N., Hino K., Ishiwata C., Kako M., Ujiie N., Endo C., Matsui A., Okamoto H., Mishiro S., "Transmission of Hepatitis C Virus from Mother to Infants." *N Eng J Med,* 1994; 330: 744-750.
9. Roberts C.M. "Genital Herpes: Evolving epidemiology and current management." *Official Journal of the American Academy of Physician Assistants,* 2003; 16: 36-40.
10. Stahelin-Massik J., Carrel T., Duppenthaler A., Zelinger G., Gnehm H.E. "Congenital tuberculosis in a premature infant." *Swiss Medical Weekly,* 1992; 132: 598-602.
11. Trijbels-Smeulders M., Gerards L.J., deJong P., vanLingen R.A., Adriannse A.H., de Jonge G.A., Kollee L.A. "Epidemiology of neonatal group B streptococcus disease in The Netherlands 1997-8." *Paediatric and Perinatal Epidemiology,* 2002; 16: 334-41.
12. Tovo Pa de Martino M., Gabiano C., Galli L., Capello N.,Ruga E., Tulisso S., Vierucca A., Loy A., Zuccotti G.V., et al. "Mode of delivery and gestational age influence prenatal HIV-1 transmission." *Italian Register for HIV Infection in Children. Journal of Acquired Immune Deficiency Syndromes & Human Retrovirology,* 1996; 11: 88-94.
13. Star J., Powrie R., Cu-uvin S., Carpenter C.C. "Should women with human immunodeficiency virus be delivered by cesarean?" *Obstet Gynecol* 1999; 94: 799-801.
14. ACOG Committee Opinion: number 279, December 2002. "Prevention of early-onset group B streptococcal disease in newborns." *Obstet Gynecol* 2002; 100: 1405-12.

SIGNS AND SYMPTOMS
OF INFERTILITY

Nothing in life is to be feared.
It is only to be understood.

—*Marie Curie*

Given the well-functioning nature of human reproductive systems, why is a certain couple having trouble conceiving a baby, or sustaining a pregnancy, or giving birth to a healthy child?

Infertile couples and their doctors understandably feel an urgent pressure to resolve this enigma. It's small wonder that they focus their attention on any obvious sign of trouble they can find: for example, an atypically low number of sperm or a thinner-than-normal lining in the uterus. Unfortunately, they often—I would even say usually—stop their investigation there and immediately begin a therapy to correct or overcome the obstacle. Low sperm count? Let's concentrate the available sperm into a specific amount of fluid and then inject the fluid directly into the uterus. Thin uterine lining? Let's use hormone supplements to create a thicker lining.

The problem with this strategy is that it confuses a sign or symptom of a problem with the source or cause of that problem. Unless the latter is tackled first, the problem will continue to bedevil repro-

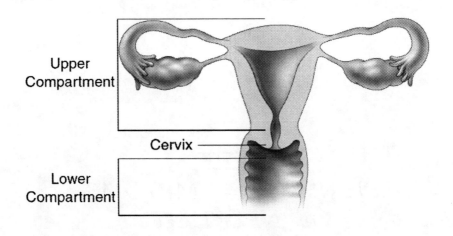

Figure 3
Schematic diagram of the female internal genital organs. Note the position of the cervix separating the upper and lower compartments.

duction, resulting in a continued failure to conceive, a troubled pregnancy, an unhealthy baby, and/or an inability to produce future children.

Take, for example, the diagnosis "low sperm count." What is causing that? If the source is an infection that is much more difficult and time-consuming to see and identify than the low sperm count in itself, working to eradicate the infection increases the chances that the sperm count can improve and conception can occur the best possible way—as nature intended. Even if the sperm count doesn't recover and it is then decided to inject the sperm into the uterus, the injected sperm will be far less likely to carry infectious agents directly into the uterine environment, where they could continue to thwart the reproductive process.

In the case of the thin uterine lining, the same logic applies. Almost certainly, the thinness is caused by infectious agents. Leaving the infection untreated or undertreated in favor of using hormone supplements right away does not remove a problem that can still cause infertility. When dealing with this situation, it makes far more sense in the long run to remove the infection first. The lining may then restore itself naturally. If it can't, hormone supplements can be used with more safety and greater odds for success.

In this chapter, we'll consider more closely the borderline state between fertility and infertility. We'll begin by examining how the male and female reproductive systems function naturally to create a baby. Then we'll look at common signs and symptoms of infertility in men and women: the problematic conditions that are most visible—at least to a doctor—and that most often become labeled as diagnoses. After that, I'll offer recommendations about when and how to consult a doctor to deal with infertility.

A Miracle by Nature: How Fertility Works

The more you understand the basics of what is supposed to happen in human reproduction, the more able you will be to discuss infertility with your doctors and to make intelligent decisions about treatments and other options. The discussion below covers the female and male reproductive systems separately and then the human reproductive process as a whole.

Fertility begins when the male sperm effectively combines with the female egg to create a human embryo. This makes the man and the woman equal partners in conception. Although this equality does not carry through to the pregnancy, which, at least from a physical standpoint, is solely dependent on the woman, the two partners share near-equal responsibility for infertility in general. As far as records can tell, infertility can be attributed to the male partner in roughly 40-45 percent of the cases that present themselves for medical attention.

Records, however, can be very misleading. They are strikingly silent or ambiguous about cases in which both partners may be responsible for creating a situation of infertility. Given the high chance that any infections present in one partner's system will be horizontally transmitted to the other partner beginning with their first sexual encounter, and given the high percentage of infertility cases involving infection, it is probably wisest not to point the finger in one direction or the other.

Before we explore what can go wrong, let's concentrate on what happens when everything goes according to nature's plan. The latter should always be our primary goal, no matter what difficulties arise.

The Female Reproductive System

As I said in Chapter 2, the female reproductive system—or genital tract—has two parts separated by the cervix: an upper compartment (the more interior one) and a lower compartment. (See figure 4.) At the inner end of the upper compartment are the two ovaries. The two fallopian tubes create a connection between the ovaries and the inner (or upper) end of the uterus. The uterus itself is lined by a mucous membrane called the endometrium. At the lower end of the uterus is the cervix. Beyond that gateway is the vagina, which opens to the outside at the labia. The reproductive function of each of these underlined components is described below.

Ovaries: Situated on opposite sides, midway within the pelvis, the two ovaries roughly resemble large almonds in size and shape.

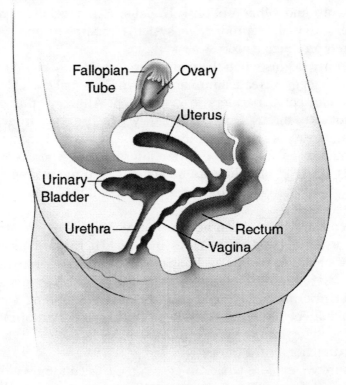

Figure 4
Lateral view of the internal female pelvis. Note the proximity between vagina and bladder. Pathogenic bacteria commonly colonize both areas simultaneously. A urinary tract infection developing during pregnancy can forewarn that an infection related pregnancy complication, such as premature labor is imminent.

From the time a woman is born, each ovary contains a fixed supply of potential eggs (also called ova; a single egg, ovum). The ovaries also generate the female hormones, estrogen and progesterone.

Each month, as part of the menstrual cycle, one of the ovaries "matures" an egg inside a tiny sac called a follicle. When the egg is fully developed, it is released from the ovary into its connecting fallopian tube.

Fallopian tubes: The fallopian tubes are narrow, two-inch-long conduits leading to the uterus. Normal fertilization—when the sperm unites with the egg—occurs inside the relevant tube. For a brief while afterward, the tube incubates the embryo. Then the tube sends it toward the uterus by means of tiny hair-like structures called cilia.

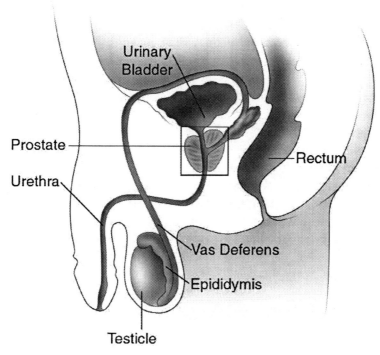

Figure 5
Schematic diagram of the male genital organs. The urethra, the lower compartment is separated from the upper compartment, seminal vesicles, vas deference, epididymis and testes by the prostate gland.

Uterus: The uterus is a muscular organ. Before pregnancy, it is roughly the size and shape of a pear, with the broad end closer to the ovaries. During pregnancy, under the influence of the abundant hormone supply produced by the placenta, it can expand up to 45 times its normal size, retaining the same basic shape, as the embryo grows into a fetus (by age two months) and then matures for seven months longer until birth. This expanding process begins when the fertilized egg emerges from the fallopian tube at the more interior end of the uterus and attaches itself to the uterine lining or endometrium.

Endometrium: The endometrium is a mucous tissue that lines the uterus. During the menstrual cycle, an escalated release of hormones causes this lining to swell with a new layer of blood vessels, providing a spongy, nutritious environment in which a fertilized egg can implant itself. If the egg is not fertilized during the cycle, or if implantation doesn't take place, this thickened layer is flushed out of the body through the menstrual flow.

Cervix: Forming the lower neck of the uterus, the cervix is a ring of muscle and collagen tissue that serves as a pivotal gateway between the uterus and the vagina. The cervix effectively separates the upper and lower compartments of the internal female genital tract. During the fertile period of the menstrual cycle, it secretes a greater-than-normal amount of mucus, favorable for sperm penetration. The dilated cervical glands serve as a reservoir that collect the sperm and then release them into the uterus. During passage through the cervix the sperm undergo capacitation, an activating process, preparing the sperm for egg penetration.

The cervix functions as both a mechanical and an immunological checkpoint. Except during the time of ovulation, sperm are kept out by the sticky mucus. Locally produced antibodies help keep infectious agents from getting through. When pathogens invade the cervix (bacterial or parasitic, such as trichomonal) the deep glands can form small, pus-filled pockets, creating a challenging problem for effective therapy. During pregnancy, the mucus thickens to form a plug. During labor, the plug dissolves and the cervix expands to allow the fetus to pass into the vaginal canal.

Vagina: The vagina is the muscular, highly elastic passageway between the uterus and the exterior surface of the body. Typically around five inches long, it is also called the vaginal or birth canal. In the lower two-thirds of the vagina, the vaginal secretion is slightly acidic. In the upper (inner) third, it is alkaline because it intermixes with the cervical secretion. During sexual intercourse, sperm travel through the cervical mucus toward the uterus. At childbirth, the vagina greatly expands to deliver the fetus from the uterus into the outside world.

The Male Reproductive System

Early in fetal development, the same core, reproductive structure starts transforming itself into a recognizably male or female system. This means that many individual features in the two systems are roughly congruent.

For example, a good look at figures 4 and 5 will provide visual evidence that the testes and the ovaries have a common point of origin in the fetus. In a later stage of fetal development, the core structure involved either remains deep inside the developing female body to become the ovaries, or it changes into testicles as a direct effect of the Y chromosome, and the testicles then descend into an exterior sac, the scrotum. Other components of the two systems also have common points of origin, although their physical similarity in side-by-side diagrams isn't as striking.

We'll return to this fact and its implications regarding infertility later. For now, let's familiarize ourselves with the major components of the male.

Testes: Also called testicles, these two oblong organs, approximately two inches long and one inch in diameter, are housed in a pouch of skin called the scrotum (or scrotal sac) that hangs outside the abdominal cavity behind the penis. This positioning gives it a slightly lower-than-body temperature internally, which is essential for its proper functioning.

The testes have two main functioning parts, the seminiferous tubules and the Leydig cells. The seminiferous tubules are the sperm-forming apparatus. The Leydig cells are interspersed between the tubules, and they produce the male hormone, testosterone. The testes produce sperm with the assistance of this hormone as well as the two main pituitary hormones FSH and LH, the same ones that initiate ovulation in women.

Each sperm is a tadpole-like cell much smaller than an egg, with a tail that can propel it through the female genital canal, hopefully to reach the egg waiting for it in one of the fallopian tubes. The testes contain no mature sperm until puberty, when increased hormonal output triggers motile sperm production. From then on, the sperm supply is in an ongoing state of replenishing itself after each ejaculation. Although a woman's ovaries form no new eggs after birth and ovulate the last one at the time of menopause, sperm production in the man normally proceeds well into the eighth decade of his life.

Epididymis: A tube coiled along the back of each testicle, the epididymis is the place where sperm continue their maturation and are stored before moving to the vas deferens.

Vas deferens: During ejaculation, mature sperm pass through the two vas deferens (one from each testicle, collectively called "vas deferens"), which are long narrow tubes running up from the epididymis and going into the prostate behind the bladder.

Seminal vesicles: The seminal vesicles are two grape-sized glands (one connected to each vas deferens) that are located behind the bladder. They secrete seminal fluid into the vas deferens to feed the sperm and lubricate their further movement.

Prostate gland: The walnut-sized prostate gland straddles the intersection of the two vas deferens, just beyond the seminal vesicles, and the urethra, coming from the bladder. Along with the much tinier Cowper's glands just below it, the prostate gland also adds fluid to enable the sperm to travel out of the male body and into the female reproductive system. The resulting combination of sperm and fluid is called semen.

Urethra: The urethra functions as the outside conduit for both urine and semen. Automatic reflexes control what goes through the urethra, so that urine is kept in the bladder during ejaculation.

Penis: The penis is a flexible, tube-shaped organ made up of spongy tissue rich in blood vessels. Sexual arousal involves nerve signals that dilate these blood vessels, causing the penis to swell and stiffen, so that it can penetrate the vagina of the female reproductive system and deliver the sperm there during ejaculation.

Conception, Pregnancy, and Birth

Even a concise overview of how a new human being comes to life inspires wonder at nature's marvelous engineering. Confronting a case of infertility, we're too inclined to think of the entire reproductive process as a fragile one. The truth is that it's amazingly well designed to work.

At the male climax of sexual intercourse, about one-tenth of an ounce of semen containing millions of sperm (the normal range is anywhere from 20 to 150 million) is catapulted into the vagina. As the sperm cells propel themselves forward with their tails, their number rapidly diminishes. Many don't survive the acidic environment of the vaginal canal. Others are unable to penetrate the cervical mucus. Only a few hundred of the strongest sperm actually reach the fallopian tubes. Even fewer sperm manage to make contact with the fertilized egg. And in most cases, only one sperm manages to penetrate it. As soon as that happens, a chemical reaction in the egg usually blocks other sperm from doing the same.

Immediately after penetration, the sperm cell and the egg cell, each containing 23 genetic chromosomes, combine their genes. The result is a transformed cell (called an embryo or, more precisely at this early stage, a zygote) of 46 chromosomes—enough to generate a human being.

The embryo then journeys into the uterus, dividing into more and more cells as it goes along. Approximately five days after ovulation, including a few days of floating in the uterus, it implants itself in the blastula stage into the endometrium. There, its upper part grows into a fetus while its lower part develops into a placenta, a tissue layer that delivers nourishment and hormones to the fetus and carries away its waste. Fetal development continues until nine months after conception, when the baby is born into the world.

For the process to work as nature intends, the following things need to happen:

- A healthy egg must be produced and released into a healthy fallopian tube that opens to receive it: activities that require the proper functioning of hormones and a clean enough environment.

- A sufficient number of well-formed, highly mobile sperm must be produced and must be able to move from the testes through the penis during ejaculation: activities that require the proper functioning of hormones and a clean enough environment.

- The penis must be able to remain erect long enough to ejaculate sperm into the vagina during the time-period of ovulation in the woman's menstrual cycle (for example, the six days in the middle of a 28-day cycle).

- A sufficient number of healthy sperm must be able to push through the cervical mucus and enter the fallopian tube holding the mature egg.

- One sperm must be able to penetrate the egg.

- The resulting embryo must be able to move through the fallopian tube into the uterus and implant itself in the endometrium.

- For the embryo to mature properly into a healthy fetus and then into a healthy baby, the uterine, cervical, and vaginal environments must remain clean enough and the woman's hormone output must remain well-balanced enough to sustain it.

THE CAUSES OF INFERTILITY

My goal in this chapter is to help you understand the major diagnoses of infertility as they are now most often announced in clinics and discussed in both the media and the medical profession. In addition, I'll extend the discussion by adding my clinical experience of thirty years regarding how infections create a fertile ground for most of these conditions. For this purpose, it makes sense to start not at the real beginning of the problems involved, but at the point where they start showing up in routine testing and ordinary conversation. First I'll describe the infertile conditions most often identified in women, and then the ones most often identified in men.

WOMEN: INFERTILE CONDITIONS

Described below are the most commonly cited causes of infertility among women. Five to ten percent of cases are diagnosed as "unexplained" because none of these diagnoses fits and no problematic situations can be detected.

Pelvic Inflammatory Disease (PID)

A third of female infertility cases are blamed on pelvic inflammatory disease that doesn't actually progress to block the fallopian tubes but instigates numerous other problems. Technically the phrase is a catchall expression for a broad spectrum of apparently similar and probably interrelated conditions, including cervicitis, vaginitis, endometritis, salpingitis (inflammation of the fallopian tubes), and oophoritis (inflammation of the ovaries). Most often in medical practice, however, the diagnosis PID is applied only to well-advanced inflammations of the upper part of the genital tract (the latter three conditions cited above). In almost all instances, PID can be traced to infectious agents. The history of my patients Lyle and Annie Kirk illustrates a typical case of PID-causing infection that was horizontally transmitted from the husband, who was very sexually active before the marriage, to the wife, who was virginal at the time. Annie developed symptoms of vaginitis and cystitis immediately following the honeymoon. When local medications didn't solve these problems, the couple came to me for evaluation.

Both Lyle's semen cultures and Annie's cervical ones revealed high levels of pathogenic contamination (Mycoplasma, Chlamydia, and anaerobic bacteria). A laparoscopy on Annie showed swollen tubes with very early signs of adhesions, even though the tubes themselves were structurally intact. My examination also confirmed a copious vaginal discharge and an inflamed cervix. In addition, Annie had recently begun feeling lower abdominal discomfort, a "bloated" sensation, and a small but distinct pain in the area of her tubes.

I prescribed intravenous antibiotic therapy (Clindamycin) for both Lyle and Annie. As a result, Annie's symptoms rapidly diminished. I then lost contact with them. Two years later, after two failed pregnancies, they returned to my lab, this time for infertility treatment to evaluate the cause of several miscarriages. The cultures for anaerobic bacteria were again heavily positive. It was evident that my earlier treatment of this infection did not deliver a sufficient amount of antibiotic for the couple to experience a successful pregnancy.

Lyle and Annie both repeated the intravenous therapy, this time accompanying it with an oral antibiotic (Flagyl). Annie also had periodic intrauterine washings (or lavages) with antibiotics (Gentamicin and Ampicillin). Later, they were able to achieve a pregnancy that did succeed, and their son is now a healthy two-year-old.

Damaged Fallopian Tubes

Approximately one-third of female infertility cases are attributed to problems with the fallopian tubes that prevent eggs from passing through. In rare instances, the tubes are blocked because of a congenital deformity that may or may not be correctable by surgery. In others, the obstacle is scar tissue associated with pelvic inflammatory disease caused by infectious agents.

Separating the subject of damaged fallopian tubes from the previous section dealing with PID, as I do here, is somewhat arbitrary. After all, tubal damage is the end result of PID. However, here we're focusing solely on the end result—one that requires the affected would-be mother to rely on assisted reproductive technology to create a baby. Not all cases of PID lead to this drastic conclusion, so a separate discussion of it is justified.

To get a better sense of how this condition can develop undetected and eventually compromise fertility, let's consider the case of Carmen and Juan Castillo, who consulted me after eight years of infertility. Neither of them had ever produced a child. However, there were numerous pregnancies in the background.

Carmen first became pregnant by a previous partner at age 18 and elected to have an abortion. Shortly before meeting Juan she again became pregnant, but the six-month-old fetus died in the uterus and was delivered stillborn. In the years after Carmen's and Juan's wedding in 1984, they achieved four spontaneous pregnancies, but none lasted longer than 22 weeks.

Tests after each of Carmen and Juan's first three failed pregnancies showed no apparent problem. After the fourth miscarriage, Carmen's doctor at the time identified an immunity problem in her blood test, so during her next attempt for a pregnancy, medication was administered to correct that problem. This pregnancy also failed. A subsequent hysterosalpingogram (HSG) showed blocked tubes.

It was clear from the day the three of us met that this case would be a candidate for IVF, since blocked tubes cannot be effectively restored to their proper function by any kind of treatment. First, however, we needed to pinpoint the reason why all the previous pregnancies were unsuccessful, and why, ultimately, Carmen's tubes became blocked. My suspicion was that a chronic case of pelvic inflammatory disease caused by bacterial infection triggered all of these problems.

I took cultures for bacteria studies from Carmen and Juan, and both sets of cultures showed a profusion of the same kind of bacteria (Actinomyces israelii). Accordingly, I put Juan on a six-week course of oral antibiotics (four weeks of Ampicillin and two weeks of Doxicycline), and Carmen on a two-week intravenous course of the antibiotic Clindamycin combined with intrauterine lavages of other antibiotics and steroids.

At the end of this combined therapy, Carmen's former antibodies greatly diminished and the bacteria cultures for both her and her husband were negative. Conception occurred during the next month with the very first IVF attempt, leading to an uncomplicated pregnancy, and, nine months later, the birth of a healthy girl.

My summary of this case is that infectious agents entered Carmen's uterine cavity either with her very first sexual partner or her first failed pregnancy. During all her subsequent fertility evaluations, this gradually progressing infection was overlooked and it lay behind all her reproductive health troubles. Even the medication given to her by another doctor for her immune problem was only a symptomatic remedy and did not address the fundamental cause. IVF was a rational solution to this case. Its success, however, was secured by the intravenous antibiotic therapy.

Endometriosis

Endometriosis is a frequently encountered gynecological condition that can lead to infertility. The term refers to the growth of the endometrium outside the uterus, a phenomenon often explained as menstrual blood flowing backward into the pelvic cavity [1]. Approximately 10 to 15 percent of women in their reproductive years have this painful condition, and it can be found in about 35 percent of women who experience infertility [2].

I personally do not believe that endometriosis exists as a separate entity. Its similarities with PID are often striking and multifaceted, and therefore I treat endometriosis as a variety of PID, caused by harmful bacteria with high autigenic potential that have gained access to the woman's uterus and internal pelvic structures [3]. These bacteria are often vertically transmitted. Anytime after menarche they can spread to the internal structures using the menstrual blood, a process that can cause endometriosis even in a sexually inactive woman. Once sexual activity begins, these bacteria can attach to sperm and thereby travel to higher pelvic structures, aggravating the condition.

Vertical transmission would readily explain the high incidence of this disease in relatives of patients with endometriosis [4]. Similarly, vertically acquired bacteria can cause identical twins to have a similar chance of developing endometriosis [5].

Both PID and endometriosis feature tissue growth-factor abnormalities, tissue inflammation, advancing adhesions, and progressive scarring. Both infections are also known to predispose the woman to develop other conditions related to the immune system, such as lupus, multiple sclerosis, rheumatoid arthritis, chronic fatigue syndrome, hyperthyroidism, allergies, and asthma. Finally, my successful experience in treating both PID and endometriosis with the same broad-spectrum antibiotics indicates to me that the two diseases, often listed separately, are, in fact, closely connected varieties of the same basic infectious conditions.

In my opinion, triple antibiotic therapy is the treatment of choice for endometriosis. Surgery is reserved for symptomatic patients with extensive adhesions or with large ovarian cysts.

For an example of a serious but not extreme case of endometriosis, let's look at the case of my patients Cilla and Russ Grimaldi and see how many similarities it bears to the case of PID that I've just recounted. Prior to their marriage, Cilla had suffered through a variety of relatively minor menstrual troubles. However, after she and Russ stopped using condoms and began trying for a pregnancy, she started experiencing more pronounced symptoms of reproductive health problems.

Cilla eventually went to a colleague of mine and complained about irregular vaginal spotting. An endometrial polyp was discovered and removed. A year later she consulted another doctor who evaluated her for persistent lower abdominal discomfort, premenstrual pain, and pain during intercourse. At that time, a laparoscopy showed early pelvic adhesions and the onset of diagnosable endometriosis. Another polyp was removed surgically and the endometriosis was cauterized.

The next year Cilla and Russ met with yet another physician, this time because of their infertility. A hysterogram on Cilla showed that a previously open tube on her left side was now completely blocked. More endometriosis tissue was removed, and Cilla was advised to stay on the birth control pill for the following six months. Her symptoms were only partially relieved, intercourse remained painful, and the couple failed to conceive a child after she came off the birth control pill.

By the time I saw the couple, Cilla was both physically and emotionally in dire straits. Her pelvic pain now ruled out intercourse altogether, and she was on disability leave from her job. Meanwhile, escalating peer pressure to have a child was making her feel more and more fearful, inadequate, and overstressed.

I had to proceed extremely carefully with Cilla's pelvic examination because of the discomfort it caused her. The tender and bloated lower abdomen was consistent in all respects with a vigorously active case of PID, so I immediately started her on a course of intravenous antibiotic therapy combined with intrauterine lavages. Later her cultures tested positive for harmful bacteria (Chlamydia), further justifying the therapy. In addition, Russ's cultures showed high levels of the same pathogen, so I prescribed a course of the same intravenous antibiotic as well as a follow-up oral course of another one (Zithromax).

Cilla's turnaround was amazing. Within ten days, her symptoms had largely abated. A month after their therapy, both Cilla and Russ tested negative for pathogens, and they resumed normal intercourse in a quest to produce a child. It took three months for conception to occur. The pregnancy went full term, and now they're the proud parents of a robust and active baby daughter.

Abnormal Ovulation

About 25-40 percent of female infertility cases are blamed on abnormal ovulation. Because hormones play such a large role in the proper formation and release of healthy eggs, most instances of abnormal ovulation are connected to hormonal imbalances. When the hormones aren't functioning well, the whole body can be affected. As a result, there may be other symptoms of this condition besides infertility, such as a chronic state of being overweight due to a sluggish metabolism.

Clinically speaking, ovulatory disorders fall into three main categories:

- The pituitary gland fails to send signals to the ovaries, so there is no menstruation. This scenario can be triggered by excessive emotional stress, anorexia, or some other nervous condition. It can also be caused by certain genetic disorders, such as Kallman's Syndrome. Typically, ovarian hormone production (estrogen and progesterone) is also low due to low pituitary production of FSH and LH.

- The pituitary and hypothalamic glands are normal. On occasion, LH hormone levels may be elevated along with testosterone levels. Patients exhibit symptoms of infrequent menstruation (oligomenorrhea) or the absence of menstruation (amenorrhea). The most common variety of this condition is the polycystic ovarian syndrome (PCO), described below.

- The ovaries themselves are dysfunctional (organ failure). In this situation, the ovaries are depleted of their follicles and eventually fail to send signals to the pituitary gland. The result is markedly elevated levels of the LH and FSH hormones, with a diminished supply of estradiol. The woman is left with physiological menopausal ovaries, or prematurely depleted ovaries, commonly caused by infections.

In my own clinical experience, I've noted that pelvic infection often leads to abnormal ovulation, and frequently the loss of predictable ovulation provides the first symptom of this infection. After all, simply because of the location of the ovaries, they cannot be considered exempt from involvement in PID.

Polycystic Ovarian Syndrome (PCO)

PCO affects between five and ten percent of women during their reproductive years and is one of the more common ovulatory problems associated with infertility. Normal ovulation is governed by a series of complex pituitary and ovarian hormone interactions. It's believed that PCO is not a distinct disease entity but rather a disease-like condition resulting from breakdowns or irregularities in this process. Infrequent menstruation (oligomenorrhea) or lack of menstruation (amenorrhea) is present in about 70 percent of PCO patients [6, 7].

PCO is a chronic condition featuring the development of cysts (rudimentary follicles) in the ovaries instead of normal, mature follicles that can go on to ovulate. Among other symptoms are elevated male hormone levels [8] and infertility. PCO can also be associated with diabetes mellitus [9], cardiovascular disease [10], endometrial cancer [11], obesity [12], and excess body hair (hirsutism) [13].

Actual cyst development is only detectable by sonogram in approximately three-quarters of PCO cases. The most common hallmarks in clinical testing are a chronically elevated level of the LH hormone and a resistance to insulin. Also, about half of the women who suffer from PCO are significantly overweight, which leads to higher levels of insulin. In some cases, ovaries enlarged by the disease can be felt during a pelvic examination.

Considering several aspects of PCO and my clinical experience, I'm convinced that vertical transmission is the best way to explain its origin. I say this because women who suffer from it also have personal health histories and family health histories that show a greater-than-normal incidence of high blood pressure, heart disease, high cholesterol levels, miscarriages, the delivery of low birth weight babies, and premenstrual syndrome (PMS) [14-19].

I firmly believe that all of these health problems can be traced to infections that have perpetuated themselves throughout the individual's life. Therefore, I also maintain that a disease that seemingly exhibits several features of genetic inheritance [20-22], is actually the result of vertically transmitted pathogens. If a woman has a sister with polycystic ovarian syndrome, she herself is very likely to have it as well, and both women run a higher then average risk of passing it along to their children. The infectious nature of this condition has been reconfirmed in my clinical practice by scores of patients who have developed identical ovarian pathology through horizontally acquired infections.

The case of my patient Selena Thompson supports the hypothesis that PCO is vertically transmitted. Selena was 25 years old when I first met her. She had been married for four years without being able to get pregnant, despite actively seeking to do so. Her personal history showed that she had experienced menstrual irregularities since puberty. Retrospective analysis of her family history told me that both of her parents had died relatively early of heart disease: her father at age 45, and her mother at age 50. Also, Selena had been an only child, even though her parents had tried to have more children after her birth.

At the time of our first consultation, Selena's periods were six months apart, and when they finally occurred, they were character-ized by heavy bleeding with large blood clots and severe cramps. She complained about excessive facial hair that compelled her to seek repeated electrolysis. A physical examination revealed male-pattern hair distribution across her abdomen and around her nip-ples as well as palpable ovaries, She was also 30 percent overweight for her height.

A pelvic ultrasound was performed on Selena. Her uterus appeared normal, but her ovaries were significantly enlarged with numerous small cysts. Lab studies revealed an elevated level of LH hormone. Both of these results, combined with her personal and family histories and her physical examination, pointed to a diagno-sis of PCO syndrome.

Based on this determination, I advised hormone therapy. It enabled Selena to get pregnant, but the baby, a girl, had to be deliv-ered by cesarean section six weeks ahead of her due date. Although the baby was small for her gestational age, she caught up in growth by the time she was two. Selena then wanted to try for another child. This was about the time I became aware of the significance of verti-cal infections.

Mindful of the difficulties associated with her first pregnancy and highly suspicious that she'd been infected by vertically transmit-ted pathogens, I ordered culture studies on her cervix and an endometrial biopsy. The findings showed an assortment of rapidly growing anaerobic bacteria. Before allowing her to try for a second pregnancy, I first put her through a course of intravenous antibiotic therapy (a combination of Gentamicin, Clindamycin, and Ampicillin). She conceived her subsequent pregnancy after much milder hormone stimulation, carried the infant to full term, and delivered vaginally a healthy, seven-pound, eight-ounce baby girl.

Today Selena's daughters are both teenagers. The older one is plump, moody, and hirsute and has a completely unpredictable menstrual pattern. A recent sonogram on her confirmed the presence of polycystic ovaries. Her younger sister is slim, even-tempered, and non-hirsute and has regular monthly periods. I reasoned that the older daughter probably received PCO-causing bacteria by way of vertical transmission, while the younger daughter did not, thanks to the antibiotic therapy administered to her mother before her conception.

Cervical culture studies of the older daughter were overgrown with anaerobic bacteria, some of which also appeared in the mother's culture studies. I suggested a five-week antibiotic therapy course for the daughter. Following three weeks of Doxicycline and two weeks of Augmentin, her period showed remarkable improvement. The pelvic discomfort and mood swings associated with the bleeding all but disappeared, and she established a more or less monthly pattern of menstruation.

I doubt that antibiotic therapy alone can always restore normal ovulation in a PCO patient. Its success lies in early recognition of the condition and prompt administration of antibiotics. As with all chronic infections, the ovarian damage in PCO patients is cumulative and irreversible. Birth control pills given to symptomatic, postpubertal women can mask a disease that should be considered both as a medical and a reproductive emergency. By the time a woman with polycystic ovaries is ready to start a family, a certain extent of ovarian damage is likely to be present, and, therefore, some form of hormone stimulation or supplementation does seem necessary.

However, antibiotic therapy is certainly beneficial in facilitating a complication-free pregnancy and in preventing the relevant pathogens from being vertically transmitted. I firmly believe that antibiotic therapy for people born with those pathogens can put them at much less risk not only for infertility, but also for infection-related heart disease, coronary artery disease, high blood pressure, diabetes mellitus, and other major illnesses.

Paradox Ovulation

Apart from the kinds of abnormal ovulation already discussed, a distinct subtype of ovulatory problems occurs in cases in which one of the fallopian tubes is blocked. Infection always spreads to the ovaries through open fallopian tubes, so when one tube is blocked early on in a pelvic infection, the corresponding ovary is shielded from further bacterial spread and is better preserved than the other ovary facing an open tube.

It is not uncommon in such situations for a woman to ovulate for several months from the ovary facing the blocked tube and then have an abnormal ovulation from the other, damaged ovary facing the open tube. The better-preserved ovary provides a larger number of eggs, can respond more readily to injected fertility drugs, and yields better eggs for ART. Paradoxically, during the course of a natural trial for a pregnancy (via sexual intercourse), those eggs cannot be transferred through the blocked fallopian tube.

Damaged ovaries

Scarring of the ovaries associated with ovarian surgery (wedge resection or resection of an ovarian cyst created by endometriosis) can also prevent proper egg development and release, resulting in female infertility. Other factors that can damage the ovaries are ruptured ovarian cysts, ruptured abdominal organs that are infected, or a longstanding case of PID. Surgical correction of scarred areas is not advisable: It leads to adhesions and problems with ovulation. The follicles fail to rupture and often turn into symptomatic cysts. Chronic ovarian pain is best managed by birth control pills. If childbearing is desired, fertility drugs leading to multiple ovulation have a chance of breaking through the scarred capsule.

Hostile Cervical Mucus

Some women cannot conceive because their cervical mucus does not enable a sufficient number of sperm to pass through. The mucus itself may be too thick, acidic, or otherwise toxic, but in any of these cases, it is characteristically sticky.

An infection is almost always the source of the problem. It interferes with glandular secretion and triggers a profusion of white blood cells, giving the mucus a cloudy, discolored look. An immune system response adds antibodies to the sticky mucus, helping it seal off the upper genital tract.

Eight to twelve hours after a couple has intercourse, using the ovulation predictor kit for proper timing, a post-coital test should be performed to check for hostile cervical mucus. The presence of a large number of highly active sperm in clear mucus indicates favorable cervical conditions. The presence of dead or sluggish sperm in sticky, cloudy mucus warrants a search for local infections and antibodies. All attempts should be made to correct the mucus by eradicating the infection with antibiotics. Intrauterine insemination should be left as a very last resort.

Incidental Causes

A small percentage of female infertility conditions can be traced to damage in the genital tract caused by a major abdominal disease, surgery, therapy (such as radiation or chemotherapy), a tumor (including a fibroid tumor), physical trauma, or drug exposure.

Congenital Abnormalities

In less then five percent of infertility cases, one of a variety of congenital abnormalities contributes to the problem. The vagina may be duplicated or absent. The hymen may require surgical perforation. The cervix may be underdeveloped or divided, in which case it may be duplicated partially or completely. The uterine body may be underdeveloped or duplicated, either partially or completely.

Some women have a condition known as "unicornuate uterus," in which part of the uterus and one of the fallopian tubes is missing. Another unusual abnormality, a "T-shaped uterus" with an incompetent cervix, is found among the offspring of women who took DES (Diethylstilbestrol), a synthetic estrogen once administered to prevent miscarriages but now banned from use. Most of the reproductive difficulty in DES-exposed women, however, is due to bacteria that were vertically transmitted from the mother—the same bacteria that caused the mother to experience her reproductive difficulty. When a congenital abnormality is associated with repeated adverse pregnancy outcomes (such as preterm delivery, breech presentation, or cervical incompetence), surgical correction is recommended.

Chromosomal Abnormalities

Only rarely are women incapable of having a baby due to a chromosomal defect. The most familiar such defect is known as Turner's Syndrome. Women with this syndrome are genetically "XO" instead of "XX." In addition to being short and infertile, they have other, variable abnormalities such a webbed neck, down-slanted eyes, and a shield-like chest. In three percent of women who repeatedly miscarry, chromosomal testing will yield some form of abnormality.

Immunological Factors

An elaborate system of cells is in charge of protecting the body from invading pathogens. Several defensive lines are in operation, sending signals back and forth about the nature and strength of the invaders. Like scouts spotting enemy soldiers, the macrophages and several other cells signal the arrival of pathogens in such a way that lymphocytes ("B" cells, arriving from bone marrow, and "T" cells, arriving from the thymus gland) develop special weapons (receptors) to attack the particular pathogens. Some of these cells will produce antibodies as ammo. Others (so-called killer cells) have specialized means of disposing of the pathogens.

These defending cells cluster around body openings, where pathogens typically gain entry. The tonsils, adenoids, and numerous lymphocytes within the wall of the gut protect the respiratory and digestive tracts. The cervix and prostate are gatekeepers of the male and female reproductive canals respectively. The marvel of this system is its ability to differentiate between the host and invading organisms.

Unfortunately, under certain circumstances, the defending cells start attacking the host, not unlike rowdy soldiers shooting randomly. The immune system starts to break down and so-called self-afflicting (autoimmune) diseases develop. The most common cause of this condition is an infection. Surface structures of invading microbes can fool the immune system and make it form self-attacking antibodies.

I look at antibodies as a secondary phenomenon caused by an infection, past or present. I believe that as early as intrauterine life, the immune system, while exposed to pathogens, can develop a hyper-reactive state, leading to asthma, allergies, and a host of other medical diseases during the individual's life after birth. It can also learn to produce antibodies against the reproductive cells or against a newly implanting embryo. When this type of situation seems to be responsible for an individual's infertility, my first step is always to test for pathogens and, if present, to offer pathogen-specific antibiotics.

In my practice, countless cases of so-called immune infertility have been successfully treated with antibiotics alone. In 15-20 percent of these couples, unfortunately, the immune problem was so strong that spontaneous reversal failed to occur following antibiotic therapy. When this happens, other forms of immune-system therapy may be the only recourse.

MEN: INFERTILE CONDITIONS

Discussed below are the most often cited problems linked to infertility among men. As with infertility conditions in women, five to ten percent of male cases are diagnosed as "unexplained" because none of these diagnoses applies and no overt problem can be detected.

Low Sperm Count

The most common diagnosis among infertile men, a low sperm count is most often unattributable to any particular cause, so it is designated "idiopathic." In the case of "oligospermia," the sperm are often not only low in number but also poor in quality: either malformed (a "morphology" problem) or poor swimmers (a "motility" or "velocity" problem). In my opinion, the cause of low sperm count and the other problems relating to oligospermia is most likely an intrauterine infection that caused damage to the testes during the man's embryonic life. As I mentioned in Chapter 2, I believe that oligospermia is the male equivalent of congenital polycystic ovaries in the female.

There is no general medical condition formally associated with oligospermia, but sperm from an oligospermic man can transmit an infection to any woman with whom he has sexual intercourse. A high percentage of cases in which both partners were previously virgins and the man is oligospermic show an apparent horizontal transmission of pathogens from the man to the woman. Among the problems the woman typically experiences are derangement of her menstrual cycle, secondary infertility, pregnancies with adverse outcomes, and recurring miscarriages. All of these conditions are reversible if both partners undergo antibiotic therapy.

Often infertility doctors use a specimen from an untreated oligospermic male for intrauterine insemination (IUI) in order to overcome a cervical mucus problem that his partner is experiencing (most likely because she acquired a horizontal infection from him). The IUI-assisted pregnancy may lead to a live birth, but it also frequently causes secondary infertility, due to the fact that the injected sperm—and the subsequent pregnancy—spread the infection throughout the woman's upper reproductive tract.

Dilated Veins around Testicles (Varicocele)

Ten to fifteen percent of infertile men have varicocele (singular or plural). These are dilated (or varicose) veins around the testes that raise their internal temperature considerably and, as a result, adversely affect sperm production. Surgery is the only option for correcting variocele itself. Since 20 percent of men with normal semen quality have a varicocele, surgery should be reserved only for those men who have significantly impaired semen quality (the actual cause of their infertility).

Damaged Vas Deferens or Epididymis

Blockage or other scar-related damage in the vas deferens or epididymis can prevent the sperm from reaching the seminal fluid. In the vast majority of cases, this problem is caused by infections. Accidental damage to these parts can occur during surgery to repair varicocele, spermatocele, or a hernia.

Hormone Deficiencies

Endocrine disorders, creating hormone deficiencies, are rare causes of male infertility. Some cases can be attributed to an insufficient or overly erratic release of the key hormones that stimulate sperm production. Specifically, this condition is called pituitary-hypothalamic hypogonadism, and it can lead to a diagnosis of oligospermia (low sperm count). Low testosterone levels and hyper-prolactinemia are associated with impotence. There is no evidence that empirically given hormone therapy benefits male fertility.

Impotence

Impotence is the inability to achieve and sustain an erection long enough to allow for ejaculation and the resulting delivery of semen into the vagina. Various different psychological issues, including performance anxiety relating to sexual intercourse, can result in impotence. Other causes include diseases (such as hardening of the arteries, high blood pressure, diabetes, or kidney disease) and environmental factors (like substance abuse or certain medications). Impotence with retrograde ejaculation (sperm enters the bladder rather then leaving through the opening of the urethra) can develop following prostatectomy or after certain cancer surgeries in the pelvis.

The recently developed drug Viagra has enabled many men to overcome impotence for a sufficient amount of time because the drug causes an artificial dilation of the blood vessels in the penis. However, certain precautions need to be taken with regard to Viagra use. It can potentially cause cardiac risk during sexual activity for men with pre-existing cardiovascular disease. It is not compatible with some prescription medications. And, in rare cases, it can cause "priapism," a painful erection lasting longer than six hours that can lead to penile injury and even permanent loss of potency.

Incidental Causes

A tiny percentage of male infertility conditions can be attributed to damage in the reproductive system caused by a major abdominal disease, surgery, therapy (such as radiation or chemotherapy), a tumor, physical trauma, or drug exposure.

Prostatitis

Prostatitis is, by definition, bacterial infection of the prostate gland. The prostate becomes the source of white blood cells and antibodies that are added to the ejaculate. An abnormal composition of this fluid can render the sperm incapable of fertilizing the egg. Inflammation of the prostate can adversely affect the volume of the ejaculate as well as the motility of the spermatozoa.

Inflammation of the seminal vesicles results in similar problems. The seminal fluid can develop high viscosity (sticky thickness). In fact, it is rare to see isolated infections of the prostate gland without the vesicular glands also being involved.

Undescended Testes

During the normal development of a male fetus, the testes form above the kidney. Later, just before birth, they descend in to the scrotum. Technically defined as "cryptorchidism," the condition more commonly called "undescended testes" is a physical abnormality in which the testes remain inside the body cavity, where the high temperature is not conducive to sperm development. Less commonly, one testicle may be present in the scrotum while the other isn't. In a small percentage of cases, undescended testes develop cancer. For this reason, surgical removal is advised.

Inguinal Hernia

Inguinal hernia, another condition associated with the descent of the testicles into the scrotum, can be characterized as complete or incomplete, unilateral or bilateral. It also is a congenital defect caused by intrauterine complications. During the development of the male embryo, chemical factors interfere not only with the migration and descent of the testicles from the abdomen but also with the closure of the abdominal wall. As a result, after descent, one or both testicles can be defective in producing sperm.

Other Congenital Defects

In rare instances, a man may be born without one of the vas deferens, one of the testicles, part of the prostate, or one of the seminal vesicles. Another rare defect is hypospadism: the opening of the urethra in an abnormal position anywhere over the lower part of the penis, a condition interfering with normal deposition of sperm in the vagina. The most common of these problems is the lack of one of the vas deferens. In this situation, normal sperm are produced but there's no duct to deliver them to the ejaculatory system. This problem can be overcome as part of an IVF—specifically, by taking sperm from the epididymis.

Immunological Causes

A number of infertile men carry sperm antibodies in their reproductive system. Under normal circumstances, sperm is effectively isolated from the immune system by the so-called blood-testis barrier. Trauma, inflammation, or a vasectomy can breach this barrier and lead to antibody formation. These antibodies, in turn, can interfere with sperm motility. In addition, antibodies covering the sperm head can hinder its ability to fuse with the egg.

In some cases, these antibodies are congenital, and in my interpretation, derived from a contaminated uterine environment. The level of these antibodies can fluctuate, and pregnancies do occur even with very high levels.

Historically, anti-sperm antibodies have been treated with steroid regimens, but today this strategy has been widely abandoned. I don't consider IUI a proven remedy to overcome infertility caused by antibodies. In cases where the level of antibodies is moderately elevated, antibiotic therapy readily results in pregnancy. If the levels are high, IVF is recommended.

Chromosomal Abnormalities

Cases of male infertility due to chromosomal abnormalities are rare. The most familiar example is men with Klinefelter's Syndrome, whose genetic type is XXY versus XY. These men are tall, mildly retarded, and always infertile.

Sperm Cell Structure Problems

Another possible, although rare, cause of infertility may be cell structure problems in sperm. Only recently have testing procedures been devised to evaluate such conditions: the DNA Fragmentation Index (DFI), which indicates the percentage of sperm cells containing damaged DNA, and the High DNA Stainability (HDS) assay, which indicates the percentage of cells with immature chromatin.

Clinical observations associate higher than 30 percent DFI and higher than 15 percent HDS with poor fertility.

GETTING HELP: WHEN, WHO, AND HOW

Often infertility is asymptomatic. In other words, an individual man, woman, or couple may not physically sense that anything in particular is wrong. However, if you do feel pain in your genital tract or notice any unusual swelling or discharge there, take it as a clear signal that you may have trouble reproducing a child. In general, any infection in the genital canal strong enough to give symptoms is stimulating the immune system and may potentially causes infertility.

Women should look out for changes in the menstrual cycle. The amount, pattern, and color of the blood, the cycle interval, and the pain associated with bleeding should not vary from month to month. Similarly, any new developments in emotional symptoms, fluid retention, or weight gain before periods warrant medical examination. For example, I occasionally see thyroid problems developing in women in response to the production of anti-thyroid antibodies. The source of these antibodies may well be a contaminated reproductive canal. For men, the presenting problem may be discomfort or difficulty associated with urination or ejaculation.

Other commonly cited indicators of potential infertility that both men and women should consider are:

- Being unable to conceive a child after three to four months. As I mention in Chapter 1, I firmly believe that medical evaluation for infertility is warranted if a couple has attempted to conceive for any longer period of time, assuming they have intercourse at least twice a week.

- Having a past history—with your current or previous partner—of infertility, miscarriage, complicated pregnancy, or children born with health problems.

- Being older than age 35.

- Having a past history of abdominal disease, infection, or injury.

In my opinion, there are many more good reasons to consult a doctor before attempting to conceive a child, if only to help ensure that there are fewer stress-triggering surprises later. In fact, the most effective time for you to begin family planning is years before you marry or try for the first pregnancy. The main reason is that you may easily have picked up one or more asymptomatic, fertility-threatening infections either horizontally or vertically or both.

It could be that such infections have never presented any symptoms to date in your reproductive history, but maybe they have manifested themselves physically in ways that you would not be inclined to connect with infertility. Perhaps they are responsible for the recurring illnesses in your early childhood. Maybe they can be linked to your parents' long struggle to conceive, or even to their bouts with heart disease. With these kinds of possibilities in mind, I've provided the questionnaires in Chapter 7 so that you can begin to assess whether you may be at high, medium, or low risk of infertility based on your background and ancestry.

No matter what your score on these questionnaires may be, or how many of the above-listed risk factors may apply to you, I urge you to consult a doctor if you have any doubt about your reproductive health or if you want to make absolutely sure that you have the best possible pregnancy resulting in the healthiest possible child.

Ideally, this consultative process is one that you and your partner should pursue as a couple. If the two of you prefer to ease into this process, you can begin by consulting a primary care physician, who can give you a broad picture of your general health and do a basic infertility workup. Whether or not you choose to see a primary care physician ahead of time—and this may be required for insurance referral purposes—by all means go to a reproductive endocrinologist (RE), who is an obstetrician-gynecologist (OB-GYN) with further training in reproductive medicine.

How do you find an RE? Your primary care physician can give you a few referrals. You can also contact the local chapter of Resolve (allied with the National Infertility Association) or local county medical societies.

As you evaluate individual referrals, carefully consider their training and background. As much as you can, communicate what you'd like to find out and what your concerns, needs, and desires are. To help you in this endeavor, you can use the information in this book along with the completed questionnaires as one basis for discussion.

Beyond everything else, remain clear and realistic about your goal and the possibility that it may or may not be achievable. Most likely what you're trying to accomplish is much more serious, joyful, and reasonable than just having a baby, any kind of baby, regardless of the cost and consequences. What you truly want is to bring a healthy baby to life, to your family, and to the world.

CHAPTER 3 REFERENCES

1. Liu DTY, Hitchchock A. "Endometriosis: its association with retrograde menstruation, dysmenorrhea and tubal pathology." *British Journal of Obstetrics & Gynaecology,* 1986; 93: 859.
2. Gruppos Italiano per lo Studio Dell Endometriosis. "Prevalence and anatomical distribution of endometriosis in women with selected gynecological conditions: results from a multicentric Italian study." *Human Reproduction,* 1994; 9: 1158.
3. Ulcova-Gallova Z, Bouse V, Svabek L, Rokita Z. "Endometriosis in reproductive immunology." *American Journal of Reproductive Immunology* (Copenhagen) 2002; 47: 269-74.
4. Sipson JL, Elias J, Malinak LR, Buttram VC. "Heritable aspects of endometriosis." In: *Genetic Studies. American Journal of Obstetrics & Gynecology* 1980; 137: 327.
5. Hadfield RM, Mardan JH, Barlow DH, Kennedy SH. "Endometriosis in monozygotic twins." *Fertil Steril,* 1997; 68: 942.
6. Franks S. "Polycystic ovary syndrome." *New Eng J Med,* 1995; 333:853.
7. Zawadzki JK, Dunaif A. "Diagnostic criteria for polycystic ovary syndrome: towards a rational approach." In: Dunaif A, et al. *Polycystic ovary syndrome.* Oxford, England: Blakwell Scientific, 1992: 377-84.
8. Ehrman DA, Barnes RB, Rosenfield RL. "Polycystic ovarian syndrome as a form of functional ovarian hyperandrogenism due to disregulation of androgen secretion." *Endocrine Reviews* 1995; 16: 322.
9. Dunaif A, SegalK, Futterweit W, Dobrjansky A. "Profound peripheral resistance independent of obesity in polycystic ovary syndrome." *Journal of Clinical Endocrinology and Metabolism,* 1989; 38: 1165.
10. Talbot E, Guzick DS, Clerici A, Berga S, Weiner K, Kuller L. "Coronary heart disease risk factors in women with polycystic ovary syndrome." *Arteriosclerosis, Thrombosis, and Vascular Biology* 1995; 15: 821.
11. Coulam CB, Annegers JF, Krans JS. "Chronic anovulation syndrome and associated neoplasia." *Obstet Gynecol,* 1983; 61: 403.
12. Insler V, Shobam Z, Barasch A, Koistinen R, Seppala M, Hen M, Lunenfeld B, Zadic Z. "Polycystic ovaries in non-obese and obese patients: possible pathophysiological mechanism based on new interpretation of facts and findings." *Hum Reprod,* 1993; 8: 379.
13. Ehrman DA, Barnes RB, Rosenfield RL. "Polycystic ovary syndrome as a form of functional ovarian hyperandrogenism due to deregulation of androgen secretion." *Endocr Rev* 1995; 16: 322.
14. Glueck CJ. Awadalla SG. Phillips H. Cameron D. Wang P. Fontain RJ. "Polycystic ovary syndrome, infertility, familial thrombophylia, familial hypofibrinolysis, recurrent loss of in vitro fertilized embryos, and miscarriages." *Fertil Steril,* 2000; 74(2): 394-7.

15. Glueck CJ. Wang P. Fontain RN. Sieve-Smith L. "Plasminoge activator activity: an independent risk factor for the high miscarriage rate during pregnancy in women with polycystic ovary syndrome." *Metabolism: Clinical and Experimental*, 1999; 48:1589-95.

16. Talbot EO, Zboroqwski JV, Sutton-Tyrrell K, McHugh-Pemu KP, Guzick DS. "Cardiovascular risk in women with polycystic ovary syndrome." *Obstetrics and Gynecology Clinics of North America*, 2001; 28(1): 111-33.

17. Devoto E. Aravena L Gaets X. "Has oligomenorrhea a pathological meaning? The importance of this symptom in internal medicine." *Revista Medica de Chile*, 1998; 126: 948-51

18. Sir-Petermann T, Angel B, Maliqueo M, Carvajal F Santos JL, Perezbravo F. "Prevalence of Type II diabetes mellitus and insulin resistance in parents of women with polycystic ovary syndrome." *Diabetology* 2002; 45: 959-64.

19. Bjecke S, Dale PO, Tanbo T, Storeng R, Erzeid G, Abyholm T. "Impact of insulin resistance on pregnancy complications and outcome in women with polycystic ovary syndrome." *Gynecologic and Obstetric Investigation* 2002; 54: 94-8.

20. Franks S. Gharani N. Mc Carthy M. "Candidate genes in polycystic ovary syndrome." *Hum Repr*, 2001; 7: 405-10

21. Franks S. Gharani N. Waterworth D. Barry S. White D. Williamson R. McCarthy M. "Genetics of polycystic ovary syndrome." *Molecular and Cellular Endocrinology*, 1998; 145:123-8.

22. Iurassich S. Trotta C. Palagiano A. Pace L. "Correlation between acne and polycystic ovary. A study of 60 cases." *Minerva Ginecologica* 2001; 534: 107-11.

CHAPTER 4

DIAGNOSING AND TREATING INFECTIONS

To raise new questions, new possibilities, to regard old problems from a new angle requires creative imagination and marks real advances in science.

—Albert Einstein

The standard, most widespread method of medically treating infertility is first to identify the problem that the patient or the patient's partner is experiencing, according to set criteria for diagnostic grouping. The next step is to work toward correcting or overriding it, again applying group-specific recommended treatment regimens.

What is wrong with this approach? Why does it so often fail to yield satisfactory results?

I believe that the fault usually lies not in the treatment phase but in the identification phase. Too many times doctors begin treating a problem as soon as they detect one, instead of investigating the problem more thoroughly to discover its root cause. In effect, they wind up organizing treatment around a symptom rather than the illness itself.

For example, suppose doctors discover that the male partner's sperm count is low. Proceeding on that information alone, they will often make a concentrated solution of sperm and inject it directly into the female partner's uterus. The truth is that the low sperm count may be due to an infection. If so, artificial insemination is very likely to transmit that same infection into the woman's upper reproductive tract, where it can wreak even more havoc.

Another example involves doctors finding hostile cervical mucus during post-coital testing of an infertile woman. Rather than investigating the cause of the poor cervical mucus, they often choose to bypass the cervical mucus altogether via artificial insemination. This rush to a solution also ends up transferring a lower genital tract infection to the uterine cavity.

In a different kind of situation, doctors may see that the hormone production is sluggish in the female partner, or they may encounter a gradually rising level of FSH (a pituitary hormone) following a series of failed IVF procedures. All too commonly they label the overall condition as "diminished ovarian reserve," because the net effect is poor egg development. Frequently, the inquiry stops right there. Hormone supplements are prescribed or stimulation regimens are doubled. However, the underlying problem may well be an ovarian or endometrial infection that could easily be aggravated by an unnatural increase in hormone stimulation.

Even if these short-circuit treatments lead to the birth of a child, they probably usher in other, very alarming consequences as well. The pregnancy and delivery are likely to be complicated. The health of the baby and the mother can be compromised. And the odds of the mother ever having another child could be drastically reduced.

What is most needed to improve the way both doctors and prospective parents deal with reproductive health problems is a set of new questions leading to new angles of observation. We must look deeper than the obvious, surface-level difficulty to find out what the real trouble is.

In the majority of infertility cases, I am convinced that pathogens are the hidden culprits, the destructive agents lurking behind the scene, the culprits we can only discover by assuming new points of view. Whether or not we know that a low sperm count, sluggish hormone production, or some other malady exists, a final diagnosis requires sharper vision. We have to shed more light on the overall problem and its background. Otherwise, we won't detect the simple but calamitous forces that all too often succeed by remaining menacingly invisible.

In my 1991 book, The Fertility Solution, I challenged the conventional perspective on infertility by stating what I'd learned to be true about pathogens after 15 years of research, testing, and practice involving over 3,500 patients annually. Through consistently examining the evidence more closely—not only slides of body fluids and tissues, but also details in the histories of my patients—I'd discovered that pathogens were the sole, direct cause of infertility in at least 50 percent of cases. What's more, I'd observed them functioning as a significant contributing or aggravating factor in most of the other cases.

This realization compelled me to advocate strongly the more widespread use of antibiotic therapy in treating infertility. At the time, antibiotic therapy was not commonly prescribed. My point of view on the matter was then considered radically new.

In the years since *The Fertility Solution* was published, things have changed dramatically. Now almost every infertility workup features some kind of antibiotic therapy. I applaud this development as a tremendous leap forward, but there remains a long way to go.

The overriding problem is that too few doctors do enough history taking and testing to establish more precisely what, where, how many, and how strong the resident pathogens are. A contributing problem is that too few doctors or clinics are qualified to do this kind of work. The professional staff members in charge of infertility therapy at a clinic often lack basic training in microbiology and infectious diseases. What knowledge they do have about reproductive endocrinology is geared toward mechanically treating hormonal deficiencies. Worst of all, the number of fully skilled laboratories that do exist is woefully inadequate.

Nothing short of incorporating microbiology as a cornerstone in the diagnostic stage will allow a full understanding of the scope of every infertility problem. Only with a multi-disciplinary approach and with a full understanding of the potential pathology, antibiotic sensitivity, and clinical significance of individual bacteria can the optimal treatment be given. In short, this kind of treatment means using the right types of antibiotics in the right amounts over the right periods of time, so that most if not all of the actual troublemakers are safely and surely eradicated.

My only regret about what I wrote in The Fertility Solution is that I did not use even bolder language to promote the greater and more intelligent use of antibiotic therapy in every case of infertility. This regret, along with all the new things we've learned since 1991 about infertility, microbiology, antibiotic therapy, and disease transmission, have motivated me to write the book you're reading now.

If Fertile vs. Infertile can be said to have a single, most important purpose, it is to urge you to seek the best antibiotic therapy applicable to your particular case of infertility. You will need to take on responsibility for the search yourself, because most doctors and clinics don't automatically guide you in that direction.

This chapter, based on my own practice, offers you guidelines and examples that will help you to discuss possible infectious problems and antibiotic solutions with any doctors and clinics that you consult. To prepare you in advance to avoid feeling confused or uninformed, it also introduces you to specific medical concerns and procedures, expressed in technical language, that may come up in these discussions.

For your convenience, the chapter is divided into two sections. Part One focuses primarily on the tricky diagnostic process: combining scientific inquiry with detective work, intuition, and common sense to determine if pathogens are likely to be causing or aggravating your infertility problem. It's an investigation in which you as the patient can play a major role, because so many clues lie in events or conditions that you alone have experienced. Part Two examines the treatment process. As you will see, this stage can be equally tricky, sometimes involving experimentation with more than one promising strategy as unanticipated barriers or setbacks occur along the way. The result, however, is often an amazingly efficient and effective restoration of reproductive capability, leading to an uncomplicated pregnancy and a healthy, full-term baby.

PART ONE—NARROWING THE LIST OF SUSPECTS: DEDUCE TO REDUCE

Thinking as a pathologist, my basic premise in evaluating all infertility conditions remains the same: extraneous agents have entered the reproductive system and caused trouble. The human body itself is designed to function wondrously well, but it is also open to contamination from the outside world. Because this kind of violation is not only the most likely cause of infertility, but also the most easily treated one, I never begin more complicated or invasive procedures for a couple until after I've completely mapped both the male and female genital canals for pathogens and then eliminated those pathogens as effectively as possible.

The mapping process does not begin with a microscope but with lists of questions, the same lists that you have in your hands (Chapter 7). Ideally, the patient and his or her partner come to my office together, and the first thing we do is to discuss these questions and their answers. Gradually and inevitably, I can see patterns develop in the personal and family histories of the two individuals: for example, recurring kinds of diseases or physical complaints, a series of increasingly difficult pregnancies, or couples with few or no children after many years of marriage. These patterns are clues that point to the probable existence of certain infertility-related pathogens now circulating in both of their bodies, thanks to the combination of vertical and horizontal transmission.

Typically this conversation lasts about an hour and a half—the most important hour and half in the entire diagnostic process. At the end of this relatively brief time, I almost always know what the couple's infertility problem is, even how it originated. Of course, I can't prove what I know on the spot, but it gives me a very good basis for deciding which pathogens to pursue when testing culture specimens taken from the patients.

As I noted earlier, testing for every possible pathogen can be expensive and time-consuming. Since antibiotic therapy, in general is by far less expensive than other infertility treatments, it is a well worth investment. Each type of pathogen requires its own, separately prepared culture. This culture then needs to be incubated for days at a time, taking up its own costly space and attention in the laboratory.

For these reasons, most doctors and clinics, functioning without the benefit of the in-depth history analysis I recommend, only do superficial testing for pathogens. Most medical treatment of infertility offered by university centers in the United States now involves some level of standardized testing for Chlamydia trachomatis, the most common and notorious bacterium. Many also have standardized testing for Mycoplasma, the next most familiar group of infectious agents. The mandatory tests performed for gonorrhea and the AIDS-related HIV virus have predominantly public health ramifications. That's where it stops.

In some cases, there is no testing at all. Instead, patients are automatically given a standardized course of antibiotics (for example, two weeks of Doxycycline) in the hope that it will eliminate any infectious bacteria that may be present. Like a shot in the dark, this form of therapy can only do a limited amount of good. Unfortunately, it also adds a new danger to the situation: an unwarranted feeling on the part of the couple and even the doctor that all infections have been knocked out, and all signals are now "go" for more complex ART procedures.

I'm convinced that a far better approach is to do a comprehensive testing for each partner in the couple. It also includes testing more than one time—especially to see if a given round of antibiotic therapy has, in fact, been successful. And it entails testing samples taken from various parts of a patient's reproductive system.

After analyzing a couple's personal and family histories, I collect physical samples for testing (both events occur during the first visit). We try to time the first visit around the time of the woman's ovulation. The ovulatory cervical mucus is then examined against the husband's spermatozoa under the microscope. This so-called ovulatory mucus-sperm slide test (OMSST) is a satisfactory substitute for a post-coital test of both fluids, which makes it a time-saver. In addition, ovulatory phase cervical mucus is the most fruitful medium to investigate when searching for the pathogen Trichomonas vaginalis.

From men, for example, I take seminal fluid to test for general bacteriology. I also obtain a swab from the urethra for chlamydia testing. If there is a question of chronic prostatitis, I also culture fluid expressed through prostatic massage and perform trans-rectal sonographic examination of the prostate gland. Scarred, enlarged areas visualized through sonography examinations are indications for direct injections of antibiotic into those areas. From women I obtain vaginal, cervical and endometrial samples for bacteria studies. The results of the endometrial biopsy will shed light on the flora of the future implantation site.

Before the visit is completed, I examine the woman's cervix with a colposcope, a low-magnification microscope, to evaluate its appearance. I look for tearing, congenital features, or anatomical defects. I also check the nature and color of the cervical mucus and any signs of chronic cervicitis. I observe the cervix again after treating it with diluted acetic acid. The painless application of this acid can bring out certain cellular features suggestive of viral infection, most notably HPV.

I also look for large ectropions. An ectropion is a folding out of the delicate lining of the inner cervical canal onto the vaginal surface of the cervix often caused by chronic inflammation. In my clinical experience, congenital ectropions are closely associated with premature or postdated birth—situations in which I suspect vertically transmitted bacterial problem.

Unfortunately, most doctors and clinics do not look closely into the different kinds of potentially problematic bacteria, at different sites in the reproductive system, that may factor into a patient's infertility. Instead, the examining physician relies simply on his or her impression of how many bacteria exist in a vaginal smear. As a result, "bacterial vaginosis" is a common catchall term among gynecologists for pathogens in general. However, the investigation can and should go much deeper, as it does in my practice. For example, if I see an infected, reddish-discolored cervix and a visibly bacteria-laden vaginal secretion, the laboratory cultures samples from both areas and antibiotic sensitivity tests are performed.

Identifying anaerobic bacteria is the most time consuming. Completing the laboratory testing can take up to three weeks. For practical purposes we don't report partial findings. In select situations, where negative cultures sharply contrast with a suspicious history, the testing is repeated free of charge.

PATHOGENS: THE CAST OF CHARACTERS

Who are the microscopic villains that can ultimately aggravate or cause infertility? In other words, who's on the list of suspects before diagnosis even begins?

The major players are commonly categorized as follows: chlamydia, the mycoplasma group, aerobic bacteria, anaerobic bacteria, parasites, viruses, and yeast.

Let's take a closer look at each of these categories individually.

Chlamydia (Chlamydia trachomatis)

During the past two decades, infection by chlamydia in the genital canal has been recognized as one of the most significant causes of infertility. Because chlamydia infection has been a reportable sexually-transmitted disease during this time period, we have a better understanding of its epidemic spread. It is now believed that up to 50 percent of sexually active teenagers acquire this infection. The Center for Disease Control and Prevention (CDC) has estimated that there are approximately four million new Chlamydia trachomatis infections per year in the United States [1].

The organism itself is an intra-cellular parasite. In other words, it's a bacterium that enters a single cell, multiplies, and eventually destroys the host cell. Once that breakdown occurs, the newly shed chlamydia organisms (which can number around 1,000) readily infect surrounding cells.

The whole process can take a few days to several months, which creates a special challenge when it comes to treatment of chronic infections [2-4]. Because antibiotics cannot reach the bacteria while it is inside a cell, they have to be kept in the patient's system until the last infected cell explodes or the infection won't be totally eradicated.

In practical terms, one can never say with certainty that a chlamydial infection has been completely eradicated. This bacterium is capable of hiding in odd cavities throughout the human body and can potentially reassert itself in the reproductive tract six months after post-therapy testing shows no trace of it. I was the first to report ovarian infection with this organism [5]. Direct visualization of chlamydia within a follicle or an ovum gives sobering credence that the infection can be transmitted vertically, which means that a newborn can carry it from day one of his or her existence.

In fact, chlamydia can travel vertically through many generations. Whether or to what extent it will surface in one generation depends on multiple factors. Carriers of the infection can then unknowingly inflict devastating damage on their sexual partners through horizontal transmission.

In the great majority of cases, an infection of chlamydia is asymptomatic. However, for a woman, a recent chlamydial infection should be suspected in any of the following situations:

- if she develops PID symptoms (such as a changing menstrual flow pattern, an onset of painful intercourse, or lower abdominal pain or discomfort);

- if she has ever been diagnosed with non-specific cervicovaginitis; or

- if a hysterogram shows blocked fallopian tubes.

Symptoms of chlamydial infection in a woman's reproductive system vary according to how deeply the organism has penetrated into the system. A recent appearance of clear vaginal secretion signals vaginal or early-stage contamination. A reduced or diminished menstrual flow, with diminishing pain as the uterine lining thins, is a sure sign of a more advanced endometrial infection. As the upper tract becomes infected and the ovaries become involved, the woman can start experiencing lower abdominal bloating and sensitivity, gas pains, irregular digestion, changes in the length of her menstrual cycle and/or ovulatory timing, ovarian cyst formation, and/or rapidly developing PMS symptoms.

In a man's body, chlamydia can be associated with non-specific urethritis. If neglected, this condition can develop into urethral stricture with restricted urine flow. Inflammation of the prostate gland can lead to acute and, later, chronic prostatitis. As the infection progresses through the epididymis to the testes, inflammation of these organs can cause painful swelling with subsequent temporary or permanent blockage of the sperm-carrying tubules.

Chlamydial infection in a man can lead to temporary or permanent reduction in sperm count or other measured sperm parameters. There is no characteristic sign in the seminal fluid for chlamydia infection [6]. However, once the man becomes infected, active spermatozoa serve as an efficient vehicle to transfer the infection to a woman during sexual intercourse. An azospermic man (zero sperm count) will infect his female partner to the level of the cervix. An oligospermic man (low sperm count) will need a longer time to cause upper tract infection in his female partner than a man with a high sperm count will. Artificial insemination with pooled, infected spermatozoa will accelerate the process.

Chlamydia's role in tubal infertility is well known. There is a strong association between ectopic pregnancy and past chlamydial infection [7]. Chlamydia can complicate the course of pregnancy and lead to miscarriages, lower birth weight, prematurity, and premature rupture of the membranes [8, 9].

Early on in my practice, while examining ovarian biopsies of patients with known chlamydial infection, I saw this bacterium in the ovaries. There's a high possibility that it can destroy the ovaries and, after a temporary, reversible phase, cause irreversible follicular destruction and ovarian failure. Let's consider the case of my patient Paula Best, who was fortunate to receive early diagnosis and prompt treatment of a chlamydial infection.

Paula was referred to me in September 1998 with a common menstrual history: she was regular until her college years, when her periods gradually became more and more irregular, skipping as many as four months at a time. The first change in her menstrual period occurred shortly after she became sexually active. By age 20, her periods completely ceased. A birth control pill regimen was instituted to keep her menstruation regular. At age 23, she married, but after a complicated and frustrating infertility workup and treatment regimen, including fertility drugs and varying procedures without a successful pregnancy, she divorced her husband when she was 32.

From 1990 on, Paula progressively suffered from hair loss, depression, and lack of sexual interest. Bone density studies showed gradually progressing osteoporosis. A year prior to her visit to our office, she was given estrogen patches, which were later replaced with Demulen birth control pills. At the time of her visit to my office, she was on Zoloft and Elavil maintenance therapy. She appeared emaciated; her height was 5'2" and her weight was 98 lbs. My examination was essentially negative. As usual, I took culture studies, and the uterine biopsy was positive for Chlamydia trachomatis.

I offered Paula a 21-day course of Doxicycline. She reported a spontaneous period a month after completing the course. Normal periods followed for the next eight months. Then she suddenly stopped having periods, and a retesting showed the presence of chlamydia again. Immediately she began a ten-day intravenous Clindamycin regimen. After the intravenous course, she spontaneously resumed menstruation and established a normal pattern.

In the middle of 1999, Paula married for the second time. Just shy of one year later, she gave birth to her first daughter. Her son was born two years thereafter.

Paula's history showed evidence of premature ovarian failure associated with a reproductive event (the beginning of sexual activity). Whenever I see this situation combined with borderline or slightly elevated FSH and LH values, I base my antibiotic recommendation on culture studies obtained from cervical and endometrial fluids as well as the male partner's seminal fluid.

Chlamydia trachomatis is not the only organism that, along with other signs, prompts me to suspect premature ovarian failure and recommend antibiotic therapy. Some of my patients with premature ovarian failure showed unusually heavy levels of, or combinations of, anaerobic bacteria in their uterine biopsy and/or their cervical fluid (and many of their partners showed the same contamination in their seminal fluid). Their menstrual cycles successfully normalized after antibiotic therapy. This happy outcome was experienced not only by patients with complete premature ovarian failure, but also by patients who were rejected from further fertility procedures or ART centers because of rising gonadotropin levels.

From the perspective of vertical transmission, one sign of possible chlamydial infection in the genetic line is early heart disease in one's own body or that of a close blood relative (grandparent, parent, or sibling), or any child born through a previous relationship. This kind of infection can also be suspected if any of the following situations have occurred:

- Either partner has been involved in a previous high-risk pregnancy requiring the management of a premature delivery.

- Either partner's mother had infertility, infectious complications prior to or after his/her delivery.

- Either partner's mother had premature menopause or documented PID before or after his/her delivery.

- Either partner's father has/had chronic prostatitis with enlarged prostate gland.

- Either partner's mother had a hysterectomy because of an ovarian cyst, irregular bleeding, or chronic infection.

Mycoplasma Group

The mycoplasma group of bacteria is very widespread in the general population.

Over a dozen family members are in the group, three definitely associated with genital tract infections and with disturbed fertility: Ureaplasma urealyticum, Mycoplasma hominis, and Mycoplasma genitalium. [10] They do their damage by coating the mucous membranes of body cavities and, in the process, adversely affecting their health and function.

Like most bacterial infections, mycoplasmal ones are often asymptomatic. For a woman, infection with mycoplasma should be suspected in unexplained infertility or recurrent first trimester losses. It can also be associated with chronic PID. In the early stages of infection, the only symptom may be a light, clear vaginal discharge, but often even that indicator doesn't occur.

For a man, symptoms of non-specific urethritis can develop shortly after mycoplasma has entered the urethra. More commonly, however, the infected male partner of a couple suffering "unexplained infertility" is completely asymptomatic. When an infected man's seminal fluid is examined, it tends to have suspiciously high viscosity and, under the microscope, the sperms show sluggish motility, with many of the sperms exhibiting fuzzy, coiled tails.

The mycoplasma known as Ureaplasma urealyticum is associated with a variety of conditions, such as infertility, spontaneous abortion, low birth weight, chorioamnionitis (inflammation of fetal membranes), urethritis, urinary calculi, and Reiter's syndrome (a response to a number of infections by the immune system in form of arthritis). Mycoplasma hominis and genitalium are linked to acute and chronic pelvic infections, which can lead to tubal infertility. They can also cause postabortal or postpartum fever and occasionally infect the newborn. [11]

In my clinical experience, mycoplasma strains that resist many drugs—and, therefore, can survive several courses of antibiotics—are the most significant offenders in infertility. I encounter numerous cases where initial therapy with both tetracycline and erythromycin fails to eradicate an infection of mycoplasma, and the laboratory test shows that the infection is resistant to these antibiotics. Also frustrating to me is the fact that the drug Zithromax sometimes fails to clear a mycoplasma infection, despite mycoplasma's "good sensitivity" to it in the laboratory (meaning that the organism typically succumbs to it).

In such situations, a stronger treatment is justified. For patients who have had recurring pregnancy losses with no apparent cause other than a persisting mycoplasma infection, I generally prescribe cyclical antibiotic therapy using doxycycline, erythromycin or Zithromax, given from day one through day ten of the menstrual cycle over three or four consecutive months. It usually leads to an uncomplicated pregnancy with delivery on the due date.

Like all other bacteria, mycoplasma can be vertically acquired from the mother's contaminated genital fluid. This fact could explain the high incidence of mycoplasma infection found among children who were exposed in their mother's reproductive tract to DES (Diethylstilbestrol, a synthetic compound prescribed in the 1950's and 1960's to prevent recurring miscarriages but later banned because the offspring exhibited reproductive problems). The infection could have originally caused reproductive failure in the mother—which, unfortunately, led to the DES prescription—and then could have traveled to the daughter, where it contributed to her reproductive difficulties.

My clinical experience suggests that if a patient's ancestral history shows reproductive difficulties that can be attributed to mycoplasma infection, then the following general rule applies: the longer amount of time that mycoplasma bacteria appear to have been in a person's family history, the stronger or more extensive antibiotic treatment is needed to eliminate it from that person's body. In other words, the most resistant strains—the ones that often cannot be completely eradicated—are derived from (at least) second- or third-generation infections.

Clues in a patient's background that an infection might have been vertically transmitted include the following:

- His/her mother had one or more miscarriages.

- His/her parents have a history of "relative" infertility: that is, one or more lengthy intervals between pregnancies during which time they failed to produce a child for unexplained reasons.

- Her mother was treated with DES. During my years of practice I have seen numerous female patients with recurrent adverse pregnancy outcomes who were never exposed to DES, and yet they exhibited the T-shaped uterus, cervical abnormalities and associated fertility problems thought to be DES-related. In such cases, I believe, the abnormalities and the reproductive failure in the offspring are not so much caused by the DES but, rather, by an intrauterine infection (commonly mycoplasma) that transfers vertically to the newborn. With every passing year, fewer and fewer DES-exposed women of reproductive age will be seen in infertility clinics.

- Either of his/her parents has/had a history of sinus trouble, postnasal drip, or chronic upper respiratory tract difficulties (mycoplasma can infect other body cavities as well as the reproductive tract). Scores of patients have reported marked improvement or complete reversal of upper respiratory tract symptoms following antibiotic therapy aimed at genital mycoplasma [12].

We routinely treat infertile patients for mycoplasma infection. In a follow-up study we conducted of patients who underwent antibiotic therapy, the group in which mycoplasma infections were successfully eradicated had a significantly higher number of pregnancies. We consider mycoplasma bacteria to be strong instigators of infertility, miscarriages, and ectopic pregnancies, especially the strains that are resistant to numerous drugs.

Aerobic Bacteria

Aerobic bacteria, as opposed to anaerobic bacteria (see below), thrive in the presence of oxygen and can be found on skin surfaces around the male and female genital canals as well as inside the canals, to the extent that oxygen is still present. They can also live around and inside the rectum.

One significant problem they can cause is called bacterial vaginosis (BV): an overgrowth of Gardenella vaginalis and associated anaerobic bacteria in the vagina. Women with BV exhibit only mild symptoms of clear vaginal discharge or no symptoms at all. The condition is more frequent in sexually promiscuous women, but a virginal woman with this condition clearly acquired the bacteria from her mother through vertical transmission. Because BV brings with it a risk of premature labor and infection of the newborn, antibiotic therapy is generally recommended during pregnancy.

I don't like to use the catchall diagnosis BV for my patients. My laboratory tests for a complete spectrum of aerobic and anaerobic bacteria and attaches a sensitivity report for each type. That means I know exactly who the offending bacteria are. Lately, group B streptococcus, Proteus species, Klebsiella, E.coli, certain staphylococci, and enterococcus fecalis have emerged as the most significant troublemakers. We often see infertility situations with stubborn vaginitis and cervical infection caused by these organisms. All too commonly, an overgrowth by these bacteria is labeled and treated as a "common yeast infection." However, a poor postcoital test is a telltale sign that these organisms are the real culprits, either by themselves or in combination with a mixed anaerobic infection.

In men, infection with aerobic bacteria such as E. coli, Proteus or Klebsiella have been seen to cause suppressed sperm motility. E. coli is known to interfere with the fertilizing capacity of spermatozoa. These bacteria have also been associated in varying degrees with acute and chronic prostatitis.

During the last few years group B streptococcus has acquired some notoriety as one of the most significant bacteria associated not only with reproductive failure but also with a series of pregnancy-related infections. The bacterium can grow under both aerobic and anaerobic conditions (the anaerobic variety is called streptococcus constellatus), which means that to achieve the optimum result, test samples need to be run both with and without the presence of oxygen in order to yield accurate results. A man can be an asymptomatic carrier of group B streptococcus. In postpartum women suffering from endometritis (inflammation of the uterus after birth), the organism is readily recovered from the vaginal canal [13, 14].

Group B streptococcus is known to be one of the chief causes of neonatal sepsis and meningitis [15]. Recently it has been associated with pre-term delivery [16]. It has also been increasingly suspected as one of the major causes of stillbirth [17] and as the key pathogen in asymptomatic intrauterine infections associated with spontaneous mid-trimester abortions [18].

During the past few years, I have observed heavy cervical and endometrial colonization with group B streptococcus in patients with histories of multiple first-trimester miscarriages. The common feature among all of these patients has been a group B streptococcal genital tract infection that persisted to a certain degree even after an initial round of comprehensive antibiotic therapy.

All of these patients went on to achieve spontaneous pregnancy within four months of the therapy. However, all of their post-conception tests showed group B streptococcus infection in the cervix. In several cases, the colonization persisted even after the administration of ten additional days of intravenous Ampicillin therapy. Following this second, post-conception round of antibiotic therapy, all of our patients carried viable pregnancies. Based on my experience with this particular group of asymptomatic patients, I'm convinced that an asymptomatic infection with group B streptococcus can affect the course of the pregnancy in any trimester, and a first trimester pregnancy loss is most likely an early manifestation of the infection.

The carrier rate for asymptomatic group B streptococcus may be anywhere from five to 40 percent of the general population [14], and there are no firm guidelines for the complete eradication or suppression of the organism. Although the ideal dose of antibiotics and length of therapy are still debated, the benefit of prophylactic Ampicillin or penicillin therapy during the third trimester is well documented in medical literature [19, 20]. Successful pregnancy outcomes for my own asymptomatic patients indicate that post-conception Ampicillin therapy and antibiotic therapy for suppression throughout the pregnancy renders such an infection harmless, assuming the natural immune responses of the patient are not strong enough themselves to do the job.

A group B streptococcus infection in the mother can also infect the neonate, which can lead to the newborn being a carrier. These individuals will harbor the bacterium without symptoms in their genital canal. When they reach puberty (and, for women, when they reproduce), the organism exerts its adverse influence. Most likely, the presence of a particularly stubborn group B streptococcal colonization in an adult means that he or she acquired the infection vertically rather than horizontally.

Without doing culture studies, I suspect that a group B streptococcus infection exists in a woman's reproductive canal if she has a history of miscarriage, especially one after the first twelve weeks of intrauterine gestation. Other indicators include a history of incompetent cervix, premature labor, premature birth with perinatal infection, and especially a newborn with an infection. It can also be associated with babies who are small for their gestational age and with sickly children who develop numerous infections in the ears, nose, eyes, or tonsils during any time period from their post-natal months to their early school years.

The complete gamut of reproduction problems caused by the group B streptococcus is represented in the case of my patient Delia Black, who visited me from the west coast for testing and later for therapy. Her personal, written account, reprinted here with her permission, speaks better than volumes of scientific publications.

I never heard of group B streptococcus until I couldn't get pregnant. Now I feel like the group B streptococcus poster girl. Although most doctors don't make a connection between group B streptococcus and infertility, miscarriage, or even pre-term birth, my unfortunate experience tied group B streptococcus to all three. Doctors often remind me that there is still little clinical research to substantiate that connection, but I have found my lay experience to be shared by many other couples.

In 1997, at the age of 32, I started trying to get pregnant. My husband and I, armed with our basal thermometer, charts, and, later, ovulation kits, wandered aimlessly down the fertility road, wondering after several unsuccessful months why it was taking so long. After eight months and much badgering, my gynecologist agreed to do some intrauterine inseminations in his office (with no drug stimulation). After four unsuccessful attempts, he finally relented and shipped me off to a fertility expert.

There, walking into the packed waiting room filled with stressed-out women checking their watches and cell phones, I couldn't help but flash to the anxious Montana cows we visited last summer who mooed relentlessly as they were corralled into the insemination tanks, dreading their turn with gloved Rancher Joe.

If I had been a cow, I literally would have been dead meat, because, after seven inseminations and more injections than I care to remember, I was nowhere. Diagnosed with undiagnosed infertility, I was encouraged to move on to in vitro. But even my in vitro experience was a bit pathetic. My husband's sperm had been tested and were willing and able to fertilize a hamster's egg but clearly wanted no part of my egg. After three days, my four eggs, which I had painstakingly grown, withered away and died in a hospital petri dish, unattended by my husband's sperm. Talk about utter rejection! I joke now, but it was sad.

Three months later, in the summer of 1998, after we took one long European vacation, I came home to discover that I was pregnant. It had happened the old-fashioned way. To say we were thrilled was an understatement. At six weeks, we looked with excitement as our little fava bean-shaped embryo's heart beat strongly. At my eight-and- a-half-week visit, I lay down with great anticipation, only to hear the words all pregnant mothers dread: 'I can't find a heartbeat.' Three days later, I ended up miscarrying. At this point, I was desperate and clung to the hope that a new doctor in New York who had helped some of my east coast friends get pregnant could help me. His name was Dr. Toth.

Dr. Toth believed that bacteria and antibodies played a role in infertility. After examining my husband and me, he found that my anaerobic culture revealed a heavy growth of Lactobacillus acidophilus. The aerobic culture showed a heavy growth of Gardnerella vaginalis. My husband, on the other hand, had Gemella morbillorum and Streptococcus constellatus, the anaerobic variant of group B streptococcus. Dr. Toth prescribed Doxicycline and Augmentin. Within four weeks, I was pregnant.

Dr. Toth's greatest concern was that if I got pregnant before all the bacteria had been eradicated, I might miscarry (my husband and I were supposed to use a condom throughout our treatment, but we cheated one fateful night). He thus continued oral antibiotic treatment for six weeks. It was a fairly normal pregnancy until 24 and one-half weeks. In June 2000, on my way to catch a flight to London from LA, I swung by my obstetrician's office because I was feeling a lot of lower pressure. Within minutes of examining me, my doctor called an ambulance. I was four cm dilated and my daughter's foot was in the vaginal canal. Our daughter died after four days in the NICU.

Going forward wasn't easy. Although most disagreed, Dr. Toth felt that group B streptococcus had been the cause of my preterm birth. I was diagnosed with an incompetent cervix. In October of the same year, my husband and I visited Dr. Toth again for another round of tests before we started trying to conceive yet again. This time he discovered that my endometrial biopsy was positive for a very heavy growth of streptococcus constellatus, the anaerobic variant of group B streptococcus. In addition, Peptostreptococcus prevotii and Propionibacterium acnes, two additional anaerobic bacteria were recovered. A heavy growth of Group B Streptococcus, an aerobic bacterium, was isolated from the cervical area. My husband's culture revealed a heavy growth of Gemella morbillorum. This time we went on 10 days of intravenous Ampicillin. Within two months, we were pregnant and resumed a ten-day course of post-conceptional Ampicillin. Even my fertility doctor was now becoming a believer.

After a cerclage, six months of bed rest, and several rounds of Penicillin VK to combat the chronic group B streptococcus infections throughout my entire pregnancy, I now have a healthy and beautiful baby girl. It wouldn't have happened without the intensive care and monitoring by Dr. Calvin Hobel and Dr. Randy Harris and advice from Dr. James McGregor. I hope to get pregnant again next year and will follow the same protocol.

As a side note: I told a friend of mine about Dr. Toth's philosophy. She had just taken her veterinary certification exam. She commented, 'Well, it makes perfect sense to me. I had to examine a mare today and discover why she was infertile. The right answer was a low-grade bacterial infection. If it plays a role in animals, then why not in humans?' Good question."

Anaerobic Bacteria

Anaerobic bacteria grow in the oxygen-deprived environments of body cavities, including the reproductive systems of both men and women [21, 22]. Many doctors fail to appreciate the significance of these organisms because they are difficult to isolate, culture, and identify due to their small individual size and sluggish growth rate.

In fact, anaerobic bacteria are probably the most important of all bacteria within the human body. Their omnipresence in the body creates a friendly environment for other bacteria and possibly other microbes, and the damaging way they can interact with the immune system makes them a prime suspect to blame for a number of immunological disorders that can lead to infertility.

In most cases, it is not a particular type of bacterium that is crucial for normal physiology to function or dysfunction, but, rather, the size of the colony and/or the variety of different species present at any given time. For example, although Lactobacillus (Acidophilus) is a normally present, "healthy" bacterium, an exceedingly heavy overgrowth can be functionally disruptive. The same is true for the anaerobes Bifidobacterium, Mobilluncus, and probably many others.

Nevertheless, certain anaerobic bacteria have recently been shown to play a more significant role in causing trouble relating to infertility: actinomyces, prevotella, capnocytophaga, and specific kinds of peptostreptococci and streptococci. Heavy growths of these organisms are occasionally found in people who are infertile or who suffer chronically infected pelvises. Mixed in with the aerobic flora of the vaginal canal, they are a potential cause of bacterial vaginosis. They have the common feature of being asymptomatic, slow growing and relatively antibiotic resistant. Because they need an elaborate oxygen-free environment for cultivation, commercial laboratories have difficulty justifying the time and labor necessary to find them.

In women, these anaerobes colonize the vagina, the cervical canal, and the internal lining of the uterus. Swabs or brushes are used to sample vaginal or cervical fluid, and an endometrial biopsy instrument is needed to collect samples from the inside of the uterus.

An excessive overgrowth of these anaerobes in the vagina and cervix—combined with a mixture of aerobic bacteria, chlamydia, mycoplasma, and yeast—is referred to as bacterial vaginosis [23]. Stubborn, recurring vaginal symptoms of this condition can emerge in the early stages of a sexual relationship. Typically the symptoms (but not the condition) either go away or become so tolerated by the woman that she ceases to notice them. During a subsequent pregnancy, the immune system is naturally suppressed, which allows these organisms to proliferate. Once the pregnancy is over, the precarious, pre-pregnancy balance between host and bacterium does not reestablish itself, and permanent vaginitis symptoms develop.

Rena Tasso's case of chronic vaginitis and subsequently developing vulvodynia well illustrates how an infection of this type develops through the course of a person's reproductive health history. At the time of our first meeting, Rena was twenty-nine years old and had been married for ten years. She wanted to investigate the cause of her progressive vaginal discomfort over the preceding year. She was convinced her husband was monogamous, as she herself was. Given the recent onset of symptoms, however, it seemed logical to assume that her husband had, after all, been unfaithful.

On the surface, this kind of case can easily be misleading. A careful analysis of every aspect of Rena's reproductive health history, however, pinpointed the origin of the infection and exonerated her husband. Both Rena and her husband are members of fertile families without a trace of vertical infection. Before marriage, however, they both were very active sexually. Rena's use of birth control was irregular and inconsistent: most often, she used the pill.

In April 1995, shortly after Rena and her husband decided to start a family, Rena experienced an early miscarriage. An ectopic pregnancy followed in June 1995, and it was managed with the drug Methotrexate, followed by a prophylactic course of antibiotics. Months later, she became pregnant again, and in May 1996, she delivered her first child, a son, close to the due date. A severe endometritis followed the C-section. She was kept in the hospital for extended intravenous antibiotic therapy.

Rena's next child, a daughter, was conceived a year later without difficulty. The pregnancy went to term. Through a normal labor process, she delivered vaginally. Her third child, another son, was conceived as planned. The baby was delivered in January 2002, through C-section, due to lack of progress and fetal distress.

Even before conceiving this third child, Ms. Tasso began experiencing vaginal discomfort. All through the pregnancy, she suffered great discomfort and needed several oral and vaginal preparations to alleviate her symptoms. Following her delivery, she endured serious postpartum depression and exacerbated vaginal symptoms.

I saw Rena one year after this last delivery. Her vaginal and cervical examination showed acute and chronic infection, and the cultures revealed a variety of heavily growing aerobic and anaerobic bacteria. It was clear to me that she had bacterial vaginosis.

Here's how I reconstruct the history of Rena's infection. The level of horizontally-acquired bacteria in her system and her husband's system was interfering with their ability to reproduce, causing a miscarriage, an ectopic pregnancy, and a poorly functioning uterus usually requiring a Cesarean section for delivery. Rena unilaterally received antibiotic therapies following her adverse pregnancy outcomes. As a result, she experienced a temporary improvement in her condition. Reinfection from her untreated husband, however, led to periodic reversals of this situation. This pattern, along with the interplay of pregnancies on her immune system, caused progressively larger colonies of bacteria to develop in her reproductive system, leading to ever more severe symptoms.

Accordingly, I prescribed lengthy intravenous and oral antibiotic therapy for both Rena and husband. It not only eliminated the vaginitis symptoms but also preserved the couple's marital life.

Bacterial vaginosis has recently received more and more attention in obstetrics. Most important, doctors and scientists have verified a significant link between excess bacteria within the vaginal canal and adverse pregnancy outcome [24]. In my own clinic, however, routinely performed endometrial cultures show that the related pathogenic bacteria are also present inside the uterine lining at the time of conception. In other words, they don't simply migrate upward to the uterus and cause trouble during the pregnancy, but are there form the beginning, possibly preventing conception in the first place.

When a woman is in a non-pregnant state, ascending anaerobic infections reaching the uterine wall will cause gradually diminishing menstrual flow. Typically, a five-day bleeding pattern becomes two or three days with brownish staining to start or finish the flow. The menstrual pain can greatly diminish. With certain aerobic bacteria (group B streptococcus) mixed into the invading group of bacteria, the flow tends to become heavier.

Most commonly, sperm carry the anaerobic bacteria beyond the cervix and contaminate the endometrium. Sadly, artificial inseminations are often the vehicle for this kind of transfer, which causes deterioration of the uterine lining. If there is no tubal blockage created by the anaerobes or a combination of anaerobes and other bacteria, the ovaries also become infected. The woman can feel the resulting damage as PMS symptoms, a reduced sex drive, less vaginal secretion, or a difference either way in cramping patterns during menstruation. Her time of ovulation shifts, and the length of her monthly cycle becomes unpredictable [25, 26].

One of the most sensitive, early signs of an ovarian infection is a gradually rising day-three FSH level. If a broad-spectrum antibiotic is promptly administered, the infection can be reversed. But if drugs are used for super ovulation to override the infection, the ovaries soon become resistant to stimulation and follicular damage results.

Internal, unfelt evidence, of anaerobic infection in a woman's upper reproductive tract includes failed ovulation and ovarian cyst formation. Chronic anaerobic infection in the ovaries can lead to chronic perio-oophoritis, commonly known as "sugar-coated ovaries" because of how the dense, surface scarring looks. This condition prevents successful ovulation. In its latter stages, it causes trapped or internal ovulation. During internal ovulation the ovaries are generating follicles in response to pituitary hormone stimulation. The ripening follicle with the egg in it reaches full maturity, but the egg is unable to break through the thickened capsule and subsequently dies off. The resulting cyst can remain in the ovary for months to come. Structures of the follicle then continue to produce the same hormones as they would during a normal cycle, and so the uterus undergoes cyclical stimulation and menstruation occurs.

Another kind of infectious condition associated with a slow-growing anaerobic bacterial infection is endometriosis. In this situation, the bacteria cause an inflammation of an internal pelvic structure. The infection spreads through the fallopian tubes to the surface of the ovaries and, following gravity, to other parts of the pelvis.

In endometriosis, a complex immune reaction develops. Antibodies form, and polymorph-nuclear leucocytes (white blood cells) go into action. A number of locally produced chemicals facilitate the adherence of shed endometrial cells to the abdominal wall, giving it the classic appearance of endometriosis.

During menstruation, every woman sheds fragments of the uterine lining backward through the tubes. Under normal conditions, these fragments are broken down by an active cell system. However, this system becomes inefficient when an infection is present. The fragments of lining are thus deposited into areas where progressive tissue damage is taking place secondary to the bacterial infection.

The presence of endometriosis is a sign of an infectious disease that responds favorably and permanently to broad-spectrum antibiotics. When endometriosis is eliminated by surgery without accompanying antibiotic therapy, the disease is likely to recur. Because of the infectious, sometimes asymptomatic nature of this condition, it can be far more extensive than the woman or her doctor may realize. Similarities in the cultured bacteria of an infected girl's vaginal secretions prior to puberty and the cultured bacteria of her mother's secretions who is suffering from endometriosis suggest that the endometriosis developing in the offspring is caused by organisms transmitted vertically, at least in the case of female offspring.

The male genital canal can exhibit the same anaerobic bacterial flora as that of the female. The pathogens can infect any part of a man's reproductive tract, and he can carry them without symptoms.

Everyone carries a certain number of anaerobic bacteria in his or her body, but medical science has not yet been able to establish what amount should be considered "normal." For this reason, the key challenge in testing is to find out how rapidly the bacteria are growing and how many different species exist. For example, although Lactobacillus (acidophilus) and Bifidobacterium species are normal bacteria within the genital tract, their heavy overgrowth will lead to a functional disturbance. The most commonly encountered anaerobes causing fertility problems in heavy overgrowth are Actinomyces, Prevotella, Bacterioides, Mobilluncus, Capnocytophaga, Peptostreptococcus, Veilonella and Streptococcus constellatus (the anaerobic equivalent of group B streptococcus).

Parasites

Trichomonas vaginalis, a monocellular amoeba, is the parasite most commonly associated with infertility. There is a 50 percent chance that sexual partners will eventually exchange the parasite, a strictly anaerobic organism that survives in a broad pH range, from markedly acidic 3.5 to alkaline 8.0. The parasite is sensitive to a drying effect in atmospheric oxygen. Therefore, once it leaves the body, it will not survive beyond a few hours.

It is believed that sexual intercourse is the most common transmission for this infection, but vertical transmission is also known to occur. Non-sexual transmission by other forms of contact is theoretically possible, owing to the organism's survival in moist secretions, but very unlikely.

Trichomonads are known for causing chronic, symptomatic vaginitis. In 50 percent of the cases involving trichomonads, no obvious symptoms occur. However, an infection can produce a yellowish, frothy cervical discharge, which, under a microscope, reveals a copious number of white blood cells and an overall granular appearance. It can also infect the cervix and the endometrium: a flagellar appendage enables it to move easily through the cervical mucus. Once lodged in the endometrium, it can prevent the lining from developing normally. In asymptomatic women, the only reliable time to take samples for microscopic diagnosis is at the time of ovulation, when seemingly copious cervical mucus washes out the flagellated trichomonads from the depths of the cervical glands. Examination on any other day of the menstrual cycle easily overlooks the non-flagellated form. The same women often exhibit trichomonads in the endometrial biopsy specimens.

Most trichomonal infections in men are asymptomatic. Some men may exhibit a mild form of dysuria or scant urethral discharge. Trichomonas vaginalis is believed to be an infrequent cause of so-called non-specific urethritis, but documenting it in the urethral smear does not prove that this organism is, in fact, the culprit. It is unusual to see complicated cases of this infection involving the epididymis and the prostate. Its toxic metabolic product is known to paralyze sperm [27].

Only recently has the role of this parasite in infertility been appreciated, and it is yet unclear whether this parasite can be held solely responsible in any one case. My clinic routinely includes testing of all infertility patients for trichomonads. Special attention is paid to patients whose ART cycles have failed in other centers as well as to patients who have poor post-coital tests or whose endometrial lining responds improperly during the luteal phase. An endometrial infection with trichomonads will adversely affect the development of the uterine lining during a stimulated ART cycle. When and if a luteal phase endometrium measured on sonography is less than 10 mm in diameter and shows poor structural development, a search for trichomonad and bacterial infections is mandatory. So far, published reports clearly show that the frequency rate of trichomonal infections among infertile couples is higher than the rate among fertile couples [28].

Viruses

HSV 2 (Herpes simplex type two) and HPV (Human Papilloma virus) are the two most commonly encountered and potentially complicating infections during the reproductive years. These two pathogens don't interfere directly with conception, but they are linked with other pregnancy-related and possibly long-term health problems.

Among women who are carriers of the herpes virus, with serum antibodies present there is no effect of recurrent clinical infection on the outcome of pregnancy. If the first infection occurs during pregnancy, the outcome can be growth retardation or premature delivery. The virus can pass through the placenta and cause infections in all organs of the baby. Severe infection acquired during the first trimester can result in spontaneous abortion.

Genital herpes infection is transmitted vertically to the newborn. If vaginal or cervical infection is documented when the baby is ready to be delivered, a Cesarean section is advised. An exposed infant should be cultured and, if needed, started on antiviral therapy [29, 30].

A well-known correlation exists between HPV infection of the female genital canal and the development of cervical cancer. Primary transmission of the virus occurs through sexual contact. Cauliflower-like lesions can affect the internal and external female genital organs and can be visualized within the male urethra. The possibility of a vertical transmission to the newborn causing respiratory papillomatosis is well documented [31, 32].

Other Possible Agents

Over the years, in a few cases, I could not find an explanation for infectious symptoms developing in a previously uncontaminated woman shortly after unprotected exposure to a particular man's seminal fluid. Although this subclass of infertility patients amounts to less than one percent of my total number of patients, every single case represented a frustrating failure.

Typically in such cases, all cultures on both partners were negative—that is, showed no signs of infectious agents. The overall picture did not indicate viral or parasitic infections: there were no allergic components in either person's system, and antibody studies were negative. Still the clinical course was always the same: once unprotected intercourse commenced while trying for pregnancy, a rapid deterioration of the entire menstrual cycle followed, with quick depletion of ovarian reserve and hormonal changes typical of resistant ovaries. Administration of fertility drugs or using IUI or IVF only hastened the development of these irreversible changes.

PART TWO

TREATING A DIAGNOSED INFECTION

As I've indicated throughout the book so far, infections acquired either horizontally or vertically are the most significant cause of infertility. This fact alone makes it logical to consider antibiotic therapy as the first and foremost treatment option for infertile couples.

In addition, other therapy options need to be postponed if at all possible until any underlying infection, the probable prime cause of the infertility in the first place, has been treated. Bypassing antibiotic therapy to engineer a birth, and, in the process, leaving the infection intact, is ignoring nature's safety filter for preventing the creation of unhealthy babies.

On a more cosmic level, it's also nature's way of averting a whole line of unhealthy human beings passing vertically-transmitted pathogens from one generation to the next, causing both infertility and a host of other significant health problems. As I discussed in Chapter 2, more and more scientists are coming to agree that ART forces not only the birth of infected children, but also the increased prevalence of major diseases in our world, including diabetes, congenital heart disease, and autoimmune health problems like systemic lupus erythematosus, rheumatoid arthritis, scleroderma, and thyroid disease.

In the past, we thought that abnormal genes were responsible for such illnesses, but we're coming to realize that the actual source is bacteria and other pathogens carried from parent to child for who knows how long (and, as a result, "masquerading" as genetic-based problems). Without antibiotic therapy, infertility treatment is a breach of evolutionary "blocking" mechanisms that are meant to keep these pathogens from wreaking their havoc [33-38].

SEVEN GENERAL RULES FOR ANTIBIOTIC TREATMENT

Before discussing individual antibiotic treatment regimens, I'd like to state seven rules that I believe apply to antibiotic therapy in general and, accordingly, to every separate case. These considerations are based on one main premise: the nine months that a human being spends in the uterine environment are the most important determinant of his or her subsequent health and future reproductive potential. That person's ensuing decades of existence outside the uterus will only marginally affect his or her basic health condition. Therefore, the fewer damaging microbes that exist in the uterine cavity during his or her gestation, the healthier life he or she will live.

Here are the seven rules that I believe all doctors and clinics, prompted by their patients, need to keep in mind when undertaking antibiotic therapy:

1. After taking a couple's histories and testing the two partners for pathogens, a course of intravenous antibiotics with uterine lavage and intraprostatic injections of antibiotics should be administered if appropriate. This treatment is advisable under any of the following conditions:

    *   If there is good reason to suspect that a pathogen was transmitted vertically. Vertically transmitted infections tend to be more stubborn.

    *   If the woman's age is close to 40 years or older and immune issues are present.

    *   If the woman has undergone a series of failed IVF cycles.

    *   If the woman has had a long history of infertility without attempting IVF but has undergone a series of failed fertility procedures, such as IUI with or without Clomid or Pergonal stimulation.

    *   If history-taking or laboratory testing shows that a woman has experienced a rapid infection-related deterioration of her ovarian function and has developed secondary ovarian failure (in fact, this situation should be considered a reproductive emergency).

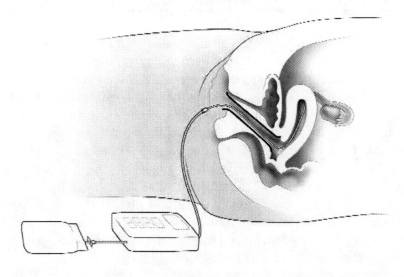

Figure 6
Antibiotic lavages of the uterus performed by the use of an ambulatory pump system and
an intrauterine catheter. Typically, one or two-hour sessions are administered during office
hours from Monday through Friday.

- If a previous child born to the woman was sickly in a way that can be attributed to vertically acquired infections or if the child had congenital defects.

In general, the intravenous antibiotic is given to both husband and wife. A continuous pump system is used to deliver Clindamycin. For the husband, this therapy is complemented with oral Flagyl and biweekly injections of antibiotics directly into the prostate gland. After the ten-day intravenous course, a follow-up regimen of oral Doxicycline follows. For the woman the intravenous Clindamycin is complemented with uterine washes using a mixture of a penicillin-type drug and Gentamycin. Local administration of these drugs avoids systemic toxicity even when used intrauterine in relatively high concentrations. Women also follow up with a Doxicycline regimen (Figures 4 and 5).

2. Err on the side of over-treating rather than under-treating. The difference can be a child without heart disease, diabetes, asthma, or a number of other adverse health conditions that he or she would otherwise acquire. If testing through proper laboratories is not available, long courses of treatment with a

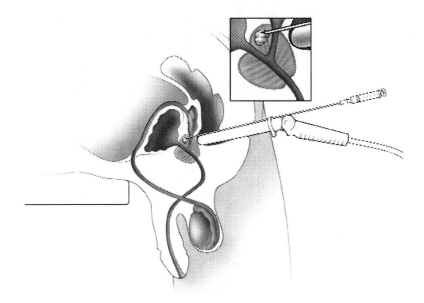

Figure 7
Transrectal, ultrasound guided antibiotic delivery into the prostate gland. Scarred, chronically infected areas are accurately targeted.

combination of broad-spectrum antibiotics should be undertaken. The proven beneficial effects of such empirical therapy (that is, treatment not based on lab results) justify it.

3. Empirically-given antibiotics should have a sufficiently broad coverage. I recommend including Flagyl to treat trichomonas, Augmentin to treat anaerobic bacteria, and Doxycycline or Zithromax to treat chlamydia and members of the mycoplasma group.

4. Always retest for the presence of pathogens following any course of antibiotic therapy. While the antibiotic is in the body, negative microbiological results are meaningless. At least three weeks should pass between antibiotic therapy and retesting.

5. Be aware of resistant bacteria and follow the sensitivity report when choosing antibiotics. This report tells you how sensitive each pathogen is to various antibiotics. You want to choose the antibiotic(s) that promise the best chance of eradicating the greatest number of pathogens.

6. Manage pregnancy aggressively with antibiotic therapy whenever it seems to be appropriate. Antibiotic therapy after conception is always indicated if a high-risk infectious situation existed prior to the pregnancy, or if the woman has a history of miscarriages, stillbirths, or long-term infertility. Therapy at this stage takes a different form so that the fetus is not adversely affected. A protocol I commonly use calls for six grams daily of Ampicillin, a broad-spectrum antibiotic, administered intravenously by a pump for ten days.

    In cases of group B streptococcus infection (according to the degree of risk and the number of pathogens that appear in follow-up testing), the patient may go on this regimen for ten days, then go off it for a month, then take oral doses of Ampicillin (500 mg) for ten more days. It may be advisable to repeat the oral therapy several times throughout the entire pregnancy.

    When the risk of infection is less severe or intravenous therapy is unadvisable, the woman can begin by taking 500 milligrams of Ampicillin three times daily orally for ten days. This therapy can then be repeated several times during the pregnancy, as required.

7. All pregnant patients should have cervical cultures at two to three month intervals during the pregnancy, including one testing two or three weeks before the birth. Regardless of whether a woman undergoes post-conception antibiotic therapy, this testing helps the obstetrician manage infection related pregnancy complications (premature labor, incompetent cervix). It helps identify pathogens in the birth canal as the baby passes through it, so that the baby can be treated, if necessary, in the most effective manner after birth.

ANTIBIOTIC THERAPY: CUSTOMIZED TO FIT THE CASE

Different infectious problems call for different antibiotic regimens. Fortunately, several of the antibiotics are compatible with each other. If a person experiences more than one kind of infection, a combined antibiotic regimen can be designed to addresses all of the pathogens either simultaneously or sequentially. For now, let's look at each problem and its solution individually.

Chlamydia

Many doctors and clinics test for chlamydia and, if present, prescribe a routine antibiotic treatment: one dose of Zithromax taken orally. In my opinion, this is woefully inadequate. I advise three weeks of Doxicycline followed by two weeks of Zithromax, both taken orally. If the patient accepts the moderate inconvenience and expense of intravenous therapy, I also prescribe intravenous Clindamycin for ten days either before or after the oral therapy.

Unfortunately, chlamydia can be elusive and it is impossible to determine what the optimum length of treatment should be in any one case because its resistance to certain antibiotics is unknown. This dilemma makes it imperative to approach each situation in the most aggressive manner possible and to retest thoroughly for the presence of chlamydia after each round of treatment. Primary sites for testing and retesting should be the cervix and the male urethra, and testing should take place both three months and nine months after therapy has been completed.

Mycoplasma

When mycoplasma is present in heavy growths either in the endometrial biopsy or in the semen specimen, I recommend an orally-administered treatment combining doxicycline and Zithromax: in many cases, 100 milligrams of doxicycline twice daily for 21 days followed by 250 milligrams of Zithromax twice daily on the first day and then once daily for the remaining 13 days. Using this regimen, my clinic has achieved a 90 percent cure rate.

When a post-therapy culture shows that mycoplasma is still present, I prescribe either Zithromax or Minocin on a cyclical basis: from day one through day ten of the woman's menstrual cycle while the couple is actively trying for a pregnancy. This regimen may continue for three to four months without interruption. The successful pregnancies achieved following such therapy tell us that mycoplasma does not have to be completely eradicated in order for a pregnancy to occur. Instead, it's sufficient to suppress them to a manageable level by keeping antibiotics in the system prior to ovulation.

Cases with a history of recurring miscarriages warrant post-conception therapy. In certain situations, we may continue throughout the pregnancy with intermittent courses of Doxicycline, Zithromax, or Minocycline. Tetracyclines and erythromycin are avoided because they entail a risk, respectively to the baby's bone and dental development.

Aerobic bacteria

The particular antibiotic therapy used to get rid of aerobic bacteria is based on the sensitivity report of the bacterium. A host of antibiotics can be used, including Cipro, Bactrim, Keflex, and Ampicillin. Vaginal cream containing Metronidazole is also commonly added to the regimen to cover anaerobic bacteria.

Group B streptococcus is the most significant bacterium in this group. I recommend especially aggressive treatment if there is a documented history of reproductive failure with pregnancy losses, premature birth, or neonatal infections in the past, short of other identified causes.

The sensitivity report for group B streptococcus most commonly suggests choosing penicillin-type drugs, Doxicycline, or Clindamycin to treat infections. In severe cases, I favor administering intravenous antibiotics combined with intrauterine washing. If follow-up testing shows that the bacterium is still present with a high colony count, I am likely to recommend cyclical antibiotic therapy until conception occurs and then intravenous Ampicillin, post-conceptionally and later oral Augmentin, or Penn Vk at intervals throughout the pregnancy: two weeks on, a month off, two weeks on, and so on.

To prevent vertical transmission of group B streptococcus infection to the newborn, if third trimester cultures are still positive, I also recommend the administration of intravenous antibiotics prior to the membrane's rupture and before the onset of labor. If the baby is exposed to group B streptococcus infection in the birth canal, there may be significant consequences. It is not uncommon to see encephalitis or meningitis develop, either of which can lead to neonatal death. This type of aggressive "forward" management of pregnancies, with intravenous therapy just prior to the birth itself, yields exceptionally good results: healthy, uninfected newborns who are much less likely to transmit a dreadful infection to their children (not at all likely if they avoid or counteract horizontal transmission before giving birth).

Anaerobic bacteria

For treating anaerobic bacteria, the most commonly effective regimen is Cleocin or Metronidazol creams applied intervaginally and, during the same time period, oral doses of Augmentin. In certain, more complicated cases, three different kinds of antibiotics are administered in the same intravenous solution: Clindamycin, Ampicillin and Gentamicin. If the endometrium is heavily contaminated with these bacteria, intrauterine washing is justified.

Trichomonads (parasite)

If cultures test positive for trichomonads, both partners take oral doses of the antibiotic Metronidazol (Flagyl) for a minimum of two weeks, 500 mg three times daily. The woman might also make regular use of a vaginal cream containing Metronidazole.

Unfortunately, Metronidazole-resistant strains of trichomonads have recently emerged. A variety of stronger treatment regimens are offered for patients who harbor these strains in their reproductive systems—for example, a combination of oral and topically applied Metronidazole. In my clinical experience, frequently suggested alternate drugs such as Paromomycin and Tinidazol have not proved effective.

I now estimate that approximately one-third of all the diagnosed trichomonal infections in our clinic are likely to resist standard Flagyl therapy. However, successful pregnancies have resulted after Flagyl therapy has been administered in cycles: both partners taking Flagyl orally for ten days—from days one through ten of the menstrual cycle again—over three or four consecutive months.

TREATMENT OF CHRONIC PROSTATITIS IN THE MALE

A recurring, frustrating phenomenon in treating male genital tract infections is that despite long courses of oral or even intravenously given antibiotic course, there remain a number of patients with persisting high bacteria counts in the seminal fluid. Persisting chlamydial infections are also a significant concern. Patients with this problem should be evaluated through transrectal, ultrasonography examination of the prostate gland. The source of the bacteria is almost always revealed as a scarred prostate lobe, abscess cavity or a markedly enlarged fibrotic prostate. In situations like this, we use transrectally-injected antibiotics directly into the prostate gland using the sonogram as a guide. The treatment was introduced relatively recently and we are very encouraged by the initial favorable results. The antibiotics selected for these injections follow microbiological findings or can be a mixture of broad-spectrum antibiotics, such as Gentamicin Levaquin and, if Trichomonads are visualized in the seminal sediment, Flagyl. If yeast infection is a concern, Diflucan is added to the cocktail. To avoid local irritating effects caused by the antibiotics, we add Xylocaine.

KATHY AND PAUL: A TRICKY CASE OF TRICHOMONADS

In some infertility cases, the absence of dramatic findings in first-visit histories or lab cultures helps point the way to the infectious culprit. It simply requires a shift in testing strategy and a more creative approach to treatment.

After being unable to conceive a child for five years, Kathy and Paul, neither of whom had ever had children, sought help at another infertility clinic. There they underwent a lengthy, elaborate, and arduous fertility workup that revealed nothing but a case of minimal endometriosis. In other words, the clinic could find no obvious reason why they couldn't produce a baby.

However, given the length of time that Kathy and Paul had tried unsuccessfully for a pregnancy, they were given a diagnosis of primary infertility and advised to enroll in an IVF program. Unfortunately, this response is standard in such situations: when in doubt, proceed immediately to the last-resort solution.

Reluctant to take such a drastic step, Kathy and Paul consulted me on the recommendation of previous patients who had subsequently had three healthy children. Nothing in Kathy's or Paul's first-visit histories or samples pointed to a specific pathogen as the culprit, which enabled me to rule out a host of infectious possibilities. The one thing I did notice was a moderately elevated level of anti-sperm antibodies on the tail sections of sperm in both of their reproductive systems. This evidence did suggest some sort of immune-system reaction to an underlying infection.

Because Kathy and Paul had never had a post-coital test, I recommended performing one during her next ovulation cycle. I knew that trichomonads, an otherwise often "hidden" pathogen frequently shows up in the ovulatory cervical mucus.

On day 13 of Kathy's next menstrual cycle, a day following intercourse with Paul, she came to my clinic for testing. The copious cervical mucus showed only a few sluggish sperm instead of the abundance of live sperm that one might expect. In addition, there were high numbers of trichomonads in the ovulatory fluid. I immediately started both Kathy and Paul on Flagyl therapy.

A month later, another postcoital test showed little difference: again only a few sluggish sperm appeared in the cervical mucus, and large numbers of trichomonads were still visible. Kathy and Paul repeated the Flagyl therapy. In addition, Kathy regularly applied commercially prepared Metrogel cream to her vagina.

The next post-coital testing revealed some improvement, but I still rated the situation "poor." Meanwhile, I'd performed an endometrial biopsy on Kathy because of her previous diagnosis of a resistant luteal phase. The biopsy sample was also loaded with Trichomonads. Putting all these facts together, I proposed injecting a Flagyl-containing preparation into Kathy's uterus. I explained that it might cause some temporary lower abdominal discomfort, but she was very willing to go ahead with the procedure if there was any chance it would help reverse her infertility.

A month later, much to everyone's delight, post-coital testing showed many healthy sperm in the cervical mucus and no trichomonads at all in the ovulatory fluid. Kathy and Paul were encouraged to try for a natural (or "spontaneous") conception. To give her ovulation a slight boost, I prescribed a hormone supplement, Clomid: 50 milligrams from day five through nine of her menstrual cycle for a four-month period.

By the end of that time, she was pregnant, and a mucus check again revealed no trichomonads. She went on to give birth to a healthy baby boy, with no maternal or fetal complications following the birth.

Six months later, after Kathy had finished breast-feeding, she and Paul tried again to have a second child. After a year and a half with no success, Kathy returned to me for a post-coital test. Sure enough, the trichomonads had come back, leaving only a few sluggish sperm in the cervical mucus. I prescribed a four-week course of Flagyl therapy for both her and her husband. With her very next menstrual cycle, she achieved her second pregnancy, which also produced a healthy baby boy.

This case brings to light several important points about treating a pathogenic infection. It proves that a trichomonal infection alone— one that may not even show up in first-visit testing—can render a couple infertile. It also shows that a given pathogen-related therapy must be tailored to fit the particular patient situation as it unfolds. Finally, it illustrates that the absolute eradication of a pathogen may not be necessary in order for the infected couple to produce a healthy baby. Instead, it is often enough simply to suppress the infection to the point that it doesn't interfere with the course of the pregnancy.

Nyla and Stan: Treating a Legacy of Problems

In some infertility situations, the strongest evidence that a particular infectious agent is to blame comes from the patient's personal and family histories and not from culture examinations. In the case of Nyla and Stan's secondary infertility, I was led to suspect a serious chlamydia infection even though initial cultures were negative for both of them. Chlamydia bacteria are adept at doing their damage in one area of the body and then hiding in another, so I knew that their failure to show up visually in large quantity on a laboratory slide (thus identifying them right away as major villains) didn't necessarily mean they weren't present in the ovaries.

Nyla and Stan flew from California to consult me before trying to conceive their first child. They were concerned about Nyla's history of reproductive health problems. Wisely, they didn't want to proceed without doing everything they could to ensure that they weren't inviting more trouble.

Nyla first began experiencing difficulties soon after an abortion she'd had in 1998, several years before she met Stan. She started skipping periods and then missing them altogether. Her doctor at the time told her that nothing could be done about it and advised her to use a birth control pill.

Nyla then went to another doctor for a second opinion. He tried a provera challenge test: the use of progesterone to initiate menstrual bleeding (appropriate in cases where the ovaries still have active follicles and produce sufficient estrogen to nourish the uterine lining). She failed this test. By then, an X-ray test showed diminished bone density, so it was decided that she should go on a course of hormone replacement therapy: cyclical administration of premarin and provera. As a result, she had been experiencing close-to-normal menstruation for three months by the time of our first visit.

Stan had no history of reproductive health problems. In fact, he'd had very few health problems of any kind from the time he was born. Although he'd had several sexual partners before his marriage to Nyla, this was his first long-term relationship. His family history was also free of trouble indicators. His parents, both of whom came from large families, had enjoyed good health all their lives and had produced three children in rapid succession before deciding to stop for economic reasons. Stan's older brother and his wife, married four years, had produced two children following uncomplicated pregnancies. His older sister, married for one year, was happily pregnant at the time.

Nyla's family history was an altogether different matter. There was no way of ignoring the possibility of a vertically transmitted infection at work in that history and, from the pattern of specific problems involved, I strongly suspected that the culprit was chlamydia.

Nyla was the younger of two sisters. Her parents had needed three years to produce her older sister, who was born one month prematurely. This child was sickly from the start and repeatedly suffered from severe ear infections and allergies. She also developed asthma early in her life and has continued to suffer from it as an adult. Four more years passed before Nyla's birth, at which time she weighed only five pounds, 10 ounces. Her mother had one more pregnancy, but the baby was a stillbirth at eight months.

The medical history of Nyla's father was also very discouraging. At age 55, he underwent triple heart bypass surgery. By that time he'd also endured numerous bouts of kidney stones: a strong indicator that an infection predisposing to stone formation could have contaminated both his urinary and the genital tracts. His two siblings, each married for many years, had both experienced secondary infertility. One had also developed prostate cancer.

Nyla's mother's history was not much better. One of her two married sisters never had children; the other, only one child in twenty years of marriage. At age 38, Nyla's mother had a hysterectomy that was prompted by a cancerous change in her cervix.

Neither Nyla's nor Stan's tested samples revealed anything out of the ordinary, although each showed a low-to-moderate level of chlamydia contamination. However, putting together what I'd learned from my own clinical experience with their family histories, I deduced that there was most likely a vertical chlamydial infection in Nyla's family. According to my reasoning, Nyla's own congenitally acquired chlamydia first gained entry to her ovaries after her very first abortion breached the barrier between the lower and upper compartments of her genital canal.

Nyla's ovarian failure qualified as a reproductive emergency, so I offered her and her husband our strongest antibiotic regimen: a ten-day course of intravenous Clindamycin. During this same time period, Nyla also underwent intrauterine lavage with Ampicillin and Gentamicin. Afterwards, they went on oral courses of doxycycline and Zithromax. The next month, Nyla reported a spontaneous period (one not assisted by hormone supplements) and complete normalization of her hormone levels. Two months later, she was pregnant, and, after an uncomplicated pregnancy, a healthy baby girl was delivered within three days of the projected due date.

Nyla's experience helped convince me that every woman who has an abortion or a miscarriage should immediately seek a careful, professional analysis of her own personal and family health histories and those of her partner. The analysis then needs to be followed by detailed testing of her and her partner's fluid samples. Taking this action is the best single thing she can do to protect her and her partner's future health and fertility, as well as the health and fertility of any child either or both of them may have in the future.

CHAPTER 4 REFERENCES

1. Centers for Disease Control and Prevention. Recommendations for the prevention and management of Chlamydia trachomatis infections, 1992. *Morbidity and Mortality Weekly Report,* 1993; 42: 1-39.
2. Dan M, Rotmensch HH, Eylan E, et al. "A case of lymphogranuloma venereum of 20 years duration." *British Journal of Venereal Diseases,* 1980; 56: 344-346
3. Campbell L.A., Patton D.L., Moore D.E., et al. "Detection of Chlamydia trachomatis deoxyribonucleic acid in women with tubal infertility." *Fertil Steril,* 1993; 59: 45-50.
4. Shepard M.K., Jones R.B. "Recovery of Chlamydia trachomatis from endometrial and fallopian tube biopsies in women with infertility of tubal origin." *Fertil Steril,* 1989; 52: 232-238.
5. Toth A., Senterfit L.B., Ledger W.J. "Secondary amenorrhea associated with Chlamydia trachomatis infection." *Br J Ven Dis,* 1083; 59: 105-108.
6. Ruijs G.J., Kauer F.M., Jager S., et al. "Is serology of any use when searching for correlation between Chlamydia trachomatis infection and male infertility?" *Fertil Steril,* 1990; 53: 131-136.
7. Cates W. Jr., Wasserheit J.N. "Genital Chlamydial infections: Epidemiology and reproductive sequelae." *Am J Obstet Gynecol,* 1991; 164: 1771-1781.
8. Gravett M.G., Nelson H.P., DeRouen T., et al. "Independent association of bacterial vaginosis and Chlamydia trachomatis infection with adverse pregnancy outcome." *JAMA,* 1986; 256: 1899-1903.
9. Martius J., Krohn M.A, Hillier S.L., et al. "Relationship of vaginal Lactobacillus species, cervical Chlamydia trachomatis and bacterial vaginosis to preterm birth." *Obstet Gynecol,* 1988; 71: 89-95.
10. Taylor-Robinson D., Furr P.M. "Recovery and identification of human genital tract mycoplasmas." *Israel Journal of Medical Science,* 1981; 17: 648.
11. Taylor-Robinson D. "Infections due to species of Mycoplasma and Ureaplasma: An update." *Clinical Infectious Diseases,* 1996; 23: 671.
12. Gurr P.A., Chakraverty A., Callanan B., Gurr S.J. "The detection of Mycoplasma pneumoniae in nasal polyps."
13. Gordon J.S., Sbarra A.J. "Incidence, technique of isolation and treatment of group B streptococci." *Am J Obstet Gynecol,* 1976; 126: 1023-1026.
14. Anthony B.F., Eisenstadt R., Carter J., et al. "Genital and intestinal carriage of group B streptococci during pregnancy." *Journal of Infectious Diseases,* 1981; 143: 761-766.
15. Pass M.A., Gray B.M., Khare S., et al. "Prospective studies of group B streptococcal infections in infants." *Journal of Pediatrics,* 1979; 95: 437-443.

16. Regan J.A., Klebanoff M.A., Nugent R.P., et al. "Colonization with group B streptococci in pregnancy and adverse outcome." *Am J Obstet Gynecol,* 1996; 174: 1354-1360.

17. Tolockiene E., Morsing E., Holst E., et al. "Intrauterine infection may be a major cause of stillbirth in Sweden." *Acta Obstetricia et Gynecolica Scandinavica,* 2001; 6: 511-518.

18. McDonalds H.M., Chambers H.M. "Intrauterine infection and sponta-neous midgestation abortion: is the spectrum of microorganisms sim-ilar to that in preterm labor?" *Infectious Diseases in Obstetrics and Gynecology,* 2000; 8: 220-2207.

19. Johnson J.R., Colombo D.F., Gardner D., Cho E., Fan-Havard P., Shellhas C.S. "Optimal dosing of penicillin G in the third trimester of pregnan-cy for prophylaxis against group B Streptococcus." *Am J Obstet Gynecol,* 2001; 185: 850-853.

20. Gilson G.J., Christensen F., Romero H., Bekes K., Silva L., Qualls C.R. "Prevention of group B streptococcus early-onset neonatal sepsis: comparison of Center for Disease Control and prevention screening-based protocol to a risk-based protocol in infants at greater than 37 weeks' gestation." *Journal of Perinatology,* 2000; 20: 491-495

21. Rosebury T. *Microorganisms Indigenous to Man.* New York: McGraw-Hill; 1962.

22. Hentges D.J. "The anaerobic microflora of the human body." *Clin Infect Dis,* 1993; 16(Suppl 3): S175-S180.

23. Hillier S.L., Krohn M.A., Rabe L.K., et al. "The normal vaginal flora, H2O2–producing lactobacilli and bacterial vaginosis in pregnant women." *Clin Infect Di,s* 1993; 16 (suppl 4): S273-S281.

24. Jacobsson B., Pernevi P., Chidekel L., et al. "Bacterial vaginosis in early pregnancy may predispose for preterm birth and postpartum endometritis." *Acta Obstet Gynecol Scand,* 2002; 81(11): 1006-10

25. Toth A. "Antibiotic therapy for luteal phase defect and premenstrual syndrome." In: *Studies in Fertility and Sterility.* Ed. Thompson W, Harrison RF, Bonnar J. MTP Press LTD. 1984.

26. Toth A., Lesser D., Naus G., et al. "Effect of Doxicycline on Pre-menstru-al Syndrome: a double blind randomized clinical trial." *Journal of International Medical Research,* 1988; 16(4): 270-279.

27. Martinez-Garcia F., Regadera J., Mayer R., et al. "Protozoal infections in the male genital tract." *Journal of Urology,* 1996; 156(2Pt 1): 340-349.

28. El-Shazly A.M., El-Naggar H.M., Soliman M., et al. "A study on Trichomoniasis and female infertility." *Journal of the Egyptian Society of Parasitology,* 2001; 31(2): 545-553.

29. Prober C., et al. "The management of pregnancies complicated by geni-tal infections with herpes simplex virus." *Clin Infect Dis,* 1992; 15: 1031.

30. Gibbs R.S., Mead PB. "Preventing neonatal herpes—current strategies." *New Eng J Med,*1991; 326: 946.

31. Schiffman M.H., Bauer H.M., Hoover R.N., et al. "Epidemiological evidence showing that human papillomavirus infection causes most cervical intraepithelial neoplasia." *Journal of the National Cancer Institute,* 1993; 85: 958-964.

32. Fredricks B.D., Balkin A., Daniel H.W., et al. "Transmission of human papillomavirus from mother to child." *Australian and New Zealand Journal of Obstetrics and Gynaecology,* 1993; 33: 30-32.

33. Aubert R.E., Ballard D.J., Bennett P.H., Barrett-Connor E., Geiss L.S., Kenny S.J. "Prevalence and incidence of non-insulin-dependent diabetes." *Diabetes in America,* 2nd ed. Collingdale, PA: Diane Publishing Company, 1996: 47-62.

34. Franks S. "Polycystic ovary syndrome." *N Eng J Med,* 1995; 333: 853-61.

35. Ehrmann D.A., Sturis J., Byrne M.M., Karrison T., Rosenfield R.L., Polonsky K.S. "Insulin secretory defects in s Polcistic ovary syndrome: relationship to insulin sensitivity and family history of non-insulin dependent diabetes mellitus." *J Clin Invest,* 1995; 96: 520-7

36. Elkayam U., Gleicher N. "Cardiac problems in pregnancy. 1. Maternal aspects." *JAMA,* 1984; 251: 2837-8.

37. American Society for Reproductive Medicine (ASRM). "Does intracytoplasmic sperm injection (ICSI) carry inherent genetic risks? A practice Committee report." Birmingham, AL: ASRM, 2000.

38. Gleicher N. "Modern obstetrical and infertility care may increase the prevalence of disease: an evolutionary concept." *Modern Trends Fertil Steril,* 2003; 79(2): 249-52.

CHAPTER 5

AFTER ANTIBIOTIC THERAPY: OTHER INFERTILITY TREATMENTS AND OPTIONS

An undefined problem has an infinite number of solutions.
—*Robert A. Humphrey*

Recently, I was consulting for the first time with a woman from California who was experiencing secondary infertility. Her repeated attempts for a second child, including several IVF procedures, had been emotionally exhausting and financially costly. Having suffered disappointment repeatedly in the past, and having never before heard about intensive antibiotic therapy, she was skeptical. "I've already invested so much in the best science has to offer," she sighed. "How could something so simple do all you claim it does? Haven't I gone beyond the stage where that kind of therapy can work?"

I empathized with her frustration. Most infertility patients must accept a great deal on faith for an indefinite period of time and simultaneously dole out large amounts of money from ever-diminishing resources. Meanwhile, the temptation to shorten the process and skip ahead to the most sophisticated scientific procedures grows ever stronger, not only for patients, but also for their doctors. In many cases, however, they give in too early or too irrevocably.

Unfortunately, this approach in solving infertility is a complete denial of the fact that infections play a critical role in causing the condition. Bypassing antibiotic therapy first is asking for failure or sub-optimal outcome.

"Do you agree with me that your child would be better off developing in a uterus that is free of infection?" I countered.

"Of course," she replied.

"Then suppose we don't do everything we reasonably can to make sure that your uterus is clean, and there is a chance for your child to develop a health problem from an untreated uterine infection. Do you want to conceive your child in a less than optimal environment?"

"Of course I do not."

That is why my primary treatment concern, before taking any other approach, is to make sure that the patient's reproductive system is as free of infectious risk as time, budget, and fortitude allow. Antibiotic therapy alone will help over fifty percent of all infertile couples to achieve a spontaneous pregnancy. If sufficient time has passed following successful antibiotic therapy and spontaneous pregnancy failed to occur, I reach out for other remedies. Among them, depending on the situation, are hormone therapy, surgery, artificial insemination, IVF, using donor sperm or eggs, or a surrogate mother.

Each of these treatments or options is discussed below. For the convenience of individual patients, I've organized the discussion below into sections that are labeled "WOMEN" and "MEN." Nevertheless, if at all possible, both partners in a couple should participate in every decision relating to any of these treatments or options. Aside from the fact that two heads generally think better than one, it's the surest way to avoid unnecessary misunderstandings, resentments, or failures in appreciation during a time that is inherently very stressful.

WOMEN

Hormone Irregularities: Diagnosis and Treatment

After the testing and antibiotic therapy during the fertility workup are finished and the reproductive systems of both partners are considered free of pathogens or anatomical problems, the woman's hormone levels are measured at three key points in her menstrual cycle. Three important hormones—the "conductors of the menstrual cycle"—are secreted by the pituitary gland: follicle-stimulating hormone (FSH), luteal hormone (LH), and prolactin. The other significant hormones, estrogen and progesterone, are secreted by the ovaries, in a close call-and-response relationship with the secretion of the pituitary hormones.

The first test occurs on day two or three of the menstrual cycle, when pituitary hormones show an early surge and start the stimulation of the new cycle. The level of the pituitary FSH and LH as well as the ovarian estrogen are measured from a simple blood test. At this point, we can get a ballpark sense of how well the ovaries are functioning by the values of these measurements. Every month one or the other ovary will assign an egg for the upcoming ovulation. FSH and LH levels above the normal range (more than 10 mIU per ml) are indicative of an ovary that is not maturing the egg properly. Specifically, the sluggish growth of the egg is not producing a sufficient amount of estradiol to signal to the pituitary that it is getting enough stimulation. The pituitary therefore is putting out even more of its hormones to elicit the right response.

The quality of the eggs can be different from month to month. Therefore it is possible in a given month to encounter fluctuating values in day three hormones as well. Another unfavorable scenario is a normal FSH on day three with an above normal estradiol value. This outcome suggests one of two things: either a "runaway" (overproducing) follicle or more than one egg responding to FSH in an ovary that has lost its regulatory ability to release only one egg each month.

Any of these abnormal signals is a bad omen for the quality of the egg. Why? As you already read in previous chapters, I attribute most cases of ovarian dysfunction—including resistance to the pituitary hormones—to senescence (aging) or pathogenic infection. Either way, the health of the egg is very likely to be compromised.

In my opinion, as you read in Chapter 1, doctors often refer to the problem as senescence of the ovaries simply because the woman is around or beyond age 40. In fact, the real culprit may be a reversible infection. Thus statistics give us a distortedly gloomy picture of a woman's natural prospects for giving birth in this age range.

Whether the reason is genuine senescence or infection, however, elevated pituitary hormone levels at this stage in the menstrual cycle are an early warning that the ovary is not healthy. In other words, one infertility problem—if not the only infertility problem—lies there.

In some cases involving women who are very near to menopause (perimenopausal), this day-three hormone test reveals another worrisome phenomenon: the initiation of more than one egg. In situations of multiple ovulations the measured blood estrogen level is understandably higher with a normal or even slightly suppressed FSH level. It's the response of a genuinely senescent ovary losing its monthly cycling regularity; as doctors often say, "rushing out eggs" [1-6]. Ovulation as early as day five of the cycle is not uncommon followed by a second ovulation two weeks later.

A higher-than-normal prolactin level on day three—or, for that matter anytime during the menstrual cycle—is another sign of trouble. Most medical authorities say that this over-secretion is triggered by a tumor (actually, a rare occurrence) or some other malfunction in the pituitary gland [7, 8]. I disagree. I am convinced that the problem actually lies in the ovary. The pituitary gland is simply reacting to the hormonal distress signal it is receiving from the ovary by producing more prolactin to compensate for the ovary. I came to this conclusion by observing normalization of prolactin levels after antibiotic therapy.

Antibiotic therapy offers a much better chance of restoring permanently normal prolactin levels than the most commonly prescribed oral medication, bromocriptine. Although doctors subscribing to the conventional diagnosis (i.e., a pituitary problem) work to suppress prolactin secretion, I aim toward restoring the ovary to health, which, in turn, almost always resolves the pituitary overproduction of prolactin.

In selected cases, blood samples are tested for thyroid hormones. It is commonly believed that sluggish thyroid function (hypothyroidism) is associated with infertility. In general, the majority of patients suffering from hypothyroidism are women and a significant number of them develop their thyroid condition following an abnormal pregnancy event, such as a miscarriage.

Although in most cases of hypothyroidism the specific cause is unknown, I'm convinced that women develop it in reaction to an autoimmune response triggered by a uterine infection—the same infection that led to the abnormal reproductive event. Thus it is not the abnormal thyroid function that leads to infertility; rather an abnormal reproductive event leads to the damaged thyroid gland that in turn produces abnormal thyroid hormones. In advanced cases of hypothyroidism, clinical symptoms unrelated to infertility necessitate treatment. Blood levels of TSH (thyroid-stimulating hormone) and T4 (thyroxin) help in assessing this condition.

During pregnancy, thyroid hormones pass freely through the placenta. This means that maternal hyper- or hypothyroidism can affect the development of the newborn's thyroid gland [9, 10]. For this reason, would-be mothers are strongly advised to get their thyroid levels checked prior to attempting conception. Women with polycystic ovarian disease may require additional hormone studies: male hormones (testosterone, DHEAS), serum insulin level, and lipid profile.

The second test of hormone levels comes in the middle of the menstrual cycle. At this time I check to see whether the pituitary gland is sending out a surge of LH to prompt the release of an egg and whether the ovary is producing the right amount of estradiol, which determines how much estrogen a mature, ready-to-release follicle produces [11].

The third measurement of hormones takes place seven days later, during the luteal or second phase of the menstrual cycle. This determines if there is a sufficient amount of the ovarian hormones estrogen and progesterone to thicken and maintain the uterine lining so it can implant and support the newly forming embryo [12]. Ten days following ovulation, I test the progesterone value: if it is more than 10 mg/ml, I know that the mother-to-be is not experiencing hormone induced luteal phase defect.

It is no longer necessary to perform an endometrial biopsy during the late luteal phase to determine if the lining is sufficiently built up. Sophisticated ultrasound machines can measure the thickness of the endometrium and evaluate its structural development.

As a rule, during infertility workups in my laboratory, I never propose hormone studies or an assessment of the luteal phase prior to dealing fully with infections. Experience tells me that nothing restores deficient endometrial development better than antibiotic therapy, which, at the same time, improves the luteal progesterone level. I also carry the antibiotic therapy to completion before looking for borderline FSH or LH values to explain a poor ovarian response to gonadotropin stimulation or before blaming anything else for a failed IVF cycle. Only if a hormone workup after antibiotic therapy shows abnormalities do I prescribe hormone stimulation or supplements.

It is fair to state that the more aggressive I've become about pursuing antibiotic therapy, the more conservative I've become about prescribing drugs during the post-antibiotic months. Again, it is clinical experience and laboratory knowledge that led me to this form of case management. Antibiotic therapy, by removing damaging bacteria, eliminates abnormal stimulation to the immune system. However, the antibodies that were already operational need time to calm down, usually six to nine months. After all, the best remedy for infertility, in my opinion, is to follow antibiotic therapy's time clock.

I never argue with time-conscious patients who decide they need to move at a faster pace, but I do make sure they understand the larger picture. If a pregnancy fails to occur during the very first month following the completion of antibiotic therapy, it only means that the chances for a pregnancy will be better the month after, and even better every month thereafter up to the ninth month. The same is not true if a pregnancy fails to occur after a fertility drug stimulated cycle without sufficient antibiotic therapy.

If a patient is determined to return to an IVF cycle following antibiotic therapy, my advice is to wait a minimum of three months prior to commencing the stimulation. Also, if a miscarriage takes place in the very first month following antibiotic therapy, I order an immunological workup and reassure my patient of a much better chance for a successful pregnancy in the following few months.

If the age factor of the woman is not too pressing, I don't interfere with spontaneous attempts at conceiving for a minimum of three months after the antibiotic therapy. During this initial three months, I am reluctant to prescribe hormone supplements even if isolated deficiencies are documented. Hormone levels tend to fluctuate cycle to cycle. Therefore, I would rather repeat an abnormal value than order replacement, stimulation, or supplementation. Only after a few months have passed do I resort, in an incremental fashion, to fertility drugs. First I use clomiphene for three months, then injectables. If those fail, I move on, with great reluctance, to IVF.

I refer to this protocol as the rule of three. Stepping up the fertility stimulation in three-month intervals allows me to ride out almost a whole year before the patient falls victim to an overly zealous IVF clinic. Without a recurring, documented hormone deficiency, I have great trouble justifying "empirical" fertility drug regimens. My clinical experience does not show any extra benefits of clomiphene in otherwise normally ovulating women, and pregnancy rates are not higher in a clomiphene-treated group than in one that did not receive any intervention, provided both groups have completed antibiotic therapy.

In cases with resistant infections, I add cyclical antibiotics from day one through day ten of the menstrual cycle to suppress stubborn pathogens. Mycoplasma, group B streptococcus, Chlamydia trachomatis, trichomonas, and actinomyces typically fall into this category.

The majority of patients who have a diagnosis of unexplained infertility achieve a pregnancy using this conservative approach. Even when the only possible approach to a pregnancy is via IVF, such as in cases of bilateral tubal occlusion or severe male infertility, the optimal time for a pregnancy to occur is six to nine months following the antibiotic therapy.

If post-antibiotic-therapy testing establishes that the woman has a significant hormone imbalance, we can take one of two treatment approaches: frontal stimulation (with or without luteal phase support) or luteal supplementation. The frontal approach, at the beginning of the cycle, stimulates the entire cycle by giving a boost to follicle formation. The latter aims to supplement subnormal hormone levels during the luteal phase of the cycle. Both approaches will increase the level of ovarian hormones, either by forcing the maturation of multiple eggs that will produce proportionately higher levels of both estrogen and progesterone for the entire cycle, or by directly supplementing borderline or subnormal amounts of estrogen or progesterone during the luteal phase.

It is not uncommon to combine both modalities in a given cycle. The combined approach is commonly used with IUI (intrauterine insemination) cycles. Using injectable fertility drugs is uniformly adopted by all IVF clinics.

There are several things a doctor needs to know about the pelvic area before administering fertility drugs. Except when preparing for an IVF cycle, it is advisable for a doctor to document through a hysterogram that at least one of the woman's fallopian tubes is open.

Added information about the pelvic area and its suitability for fertility drugs can be obtained through a sonohysterogram, a procedure in which saline solution is injected into the uterine cavity during an ultrasound examination. Another valuable source of information is a hysteroscopy, a procedure done under general anesthesia using fiberoptic tools for direct visualization of the inside of the uterus. The most detailed understanding of all can be obtained by means of a laparoscopy, an in-hospital procedure that features direct visualization of the internal pelvic organs through an optic instrument.

As a sequel to a pelvic infection, a woman's two fallopian tubes tend to deteriorate at different rates. One may become blocked early on in the process while the other remains open. The ovary sitting behind the blocked tube is always better preserved as it is shielded from additional bacteria that would be arriving with the sperm if the tubes were open. This can lead to "paradox ovulation," when better-quality follicles released from the sheltered ovary allow some cycles to function well and others not. Unfortunately, the ovulated eggs are unavailable for fertilization, except via IVF. In my clinical experience, the sheltered ovary responds more readily even with fertility drug stimulation, and we have learned through IVF cycles that eggs harvested from that ovary show better quality.

Following structural assessment of the tubes, a semen analysis is performed to rule out severe male-factor infertility, such as a sperm count that is too low or a very high number of abnormal sperm. Either of these conditions would make the chance for a spontaneous pregnancy remote.

Finally, an immunological evaluation is performed to make sure that there is not a high concentration of antisperm antibodies. Antibodies attached to sperm tails can effectively prevent sperm from traveling through the female genital canal. Antibodies attached to sperm heads can prevent sperm from penetrating the egg to fertilize it. A high sperm count compensates for immunological infertility better than a very low sperm count (oligospermia) does: the level of the antibodies can fluctuate and may not be high enough to damage all sperm if the sperm count is high. Amazingly, only a few undamaged sperms are needed to allow the reproductive process to proceed to fertilization.

Assuming that the tubes are open, no male-factor infertility exists, and antisperm antibody levels are not high enough to cause problems, I can jump-start the cycle by stimulating the first half of it, the so-called follicular phase. This is the frontal stimulation approach I mentioned earlier. The stimulation starts anywhere from day two to day five of the woman's menstrual cycle. Each day for the next five to seven days, she takes clomiphene (in most cases, 50 milligrams of clomiphene daily to start, with a gradual increase to 150 mg daily as a maximum dosage). Clomiphene stimulates the pituitary gland to produce more FSH and LH, and that action in turn forces the ovaries to mature more than one follicle, causing proportionately higher levels of ovarian hormones within the system. Using the lowest dose of clomiphene, two follicles at best may mature, but usually only one does.

Over-stimulation with clomiphene is very rare but still possible. Before repeating clomiphene in the following cycle, an ultrasound examination should be performed to rule out the presence of a residual ovarian cyst. It is important to look for untoward side effects of clomiphene on the uterine lining or on the cervical mucus. With good follicular maturation, an endometrial thickness less then 10 mm is cause for concern. A post-coital test should be performed during the first stimulated month to rule out an unfavorable effect of clomiphene on the cervical mucus. To compensate for these side effects, it is not uncommon to add estrogen during the follicular phase and progesterone supplementation during the luteal phase of a clomiphene regimen. Artificial insemination is sometimes indicated to bypass a clomiphene-induced poor cervical mucus.

In some instances, clomiphene is combined with HCG (human chorionic gonadotropin), which helps complete the maturation of the follicle and triggers the release of the egg. A daily intake of 100 or even 150 milligrams of clomiphene (two to three tablets) can cause significant headaches and may limit the length of therapy.

In select situations, clomiphene is used to introduce injectable fertility drug stimulation. The appropriate dose, timing, and length of the stimulation differs from individual to individual. For this reason, a retrospective analysis of a woman's response in previous cycles helps in planning the stimulation protocol for subsequent cycles.

Supporting the second half of the cycle (luteal phase), the later supplementation approach I mentioned earlier aims to compensate for documented or suspected hormone deficiencies during the second 14 days of the menstrual cycle. Most commonly, progesterone is administered in the form of medroxiprogesterone by way of vaginal cream, inserts (compounded by a local pharmacy in 100 mg or 200 mg doses) or commercially available progesterone-in-oil injections

(50 mg/ ml for intramuscular use). Some IUI and all IVF protocols call for progesterone support. Select IVF protocols add estrogen to the progesterone regimen (Estrace, 0.5, 1.0 or 2.0 mg daily oral tablets) Support of the second half of the cycle typically starts on the day of ovulation or on the day of follicular aspiration during an IVF cycle.

The approach I choose, frontal or later, is different from patient to patient because it needs to fit the specific demands of the situation. It's not always wise to start interfering with the natural process at the beginning of the cycle or to intervene only during the luteal phase. Again, my approach toward using fertility drugs is conservative and I recommend that approach for the profession as a whole. As I outlined above, I prefer to schedule post-antibiotic infertility therapy according to the rule of three: three consecutive three-month periods, during which patients start with no medical intervention and then undergo progressively more advanced forms of treatment in each period. This timetable gives patients the best chance of conceiving with the least amount of fertility drug stimulation. It also helps the immune system to recover and gives the doctor more time to fine-tune the process and follow the patient's incremental responses.

Moving on to injectable hormone therapy requires several considerations. The drugs are expensive. Even more important, the would-be parents may be too emotionally drained by this time to go through another three-month round of attempts. They've already endured six cycles in a row of hoping, waiting, and failing to produce a pregnancy.

Assuming these matters don't present insurmountable obstacles, injectable therapy is the most logical next course of action. It may well be the one remaining step needed to achieve a pregnancy. If so, the couple won't have to engage in riskier and more expensive IVF, or consider surrogacy, or abandon their dream of producing their own baby.

Injectable therapy starts with daily intramuscular shots of either pure FSH (Follistim, Gonal F) or a mixture of FSH and LH (Pergonal, Repronex). The usual 10-day course begins on day three of the menstrual cycle. If successful, it will typically cause the development of a multitude of follicles, with the well-appreciated possibility of overstimulation in some cases. All cycles using injectable fertility drugs need to be monitored with both serial blood estrogen measurements and serial assessment of the follicular growth with ultrasound. An

HCG injection then triggers the release of the eggs. Since there is an increased chance for multiple births, all attempts should be made to avoid high order pregnancies (13).

After the eggs are released, there are two possible scenarios. Assuming the cervical mucus is confirmed as clear—favorable for sperm penetration by a post-coital test—the couple goes on to try for a spontaneous conception. If the mucus is not clear and can't be corrected, the only choice is artificial insemination: two times, a day apart, washed, purified and concentrated sperm are injected directly into the uterus.

Meanwhile, in either scenario, progesterone is administered to support the luteal phase of the menstrual cycle (the specific protocols are outlined above). This support has to be monitored with blood progesterone measurements and adjusted if necessary. Ten days after release of the eggs or artificial insemination (depending on the scenario), the woman takes a pregnancy test. If it's negative, the progesterone supplementation is stopped. If it's positive, progesterone can be administered continuously for several more weeks until satisfactory fetal development is documented with ultrasound.

Injectable therapy may involve pretreatment with a few days of clomiphene. In fact, various drug regimens, customized to suit the individual patient, can be used to achieve optimal results. Some patients respond better to pure FSH-type drugs, while others do better with drugs that combine FSH and LH. Patients may benefit from pretreatment with a few months of birth control pills or a longer or shorter course of lupron to calm down or "deregulate" the ovaries, thus allowing multiple eggs of the same age to mature.

A woman needs to be certain she's emotionally prepared to go through with the added complications and challenges of hormone treatment. In addition to causing more physical stress, excess hormones created by these drugs can generate more emotional stress. Any woman who chooses to take this route will need even more support from her partner and her physician. Also, the more she can do to ensure that her life as a whole won't be overly demanding while she's pursuing this kind of treatment, the better it will be for her personally and for her chances to conceive.

If a woman is over age 40, time constraints on her natural years of fertility usually make it appropriate to suspend the rule of three altogether and, instead, use only the more advanced approaches over a shorter period of time. The same strategy is advisable for women who have a history studded with numerous reproductive problems and failed fertility treatment regimens, such as multiple failed IVF cycles. For these patients following antibiotic therapy, it is not smart or kind to recommend three months of trying for a spontaneous or medically unassisted conception. They typically understand the limitations of their situation. Because of their longer history of coping with infertility treatments, they tend to be well informed about the subject, active in support groups providing not only counsel but also emotional reinforcement, and committed to their own agenda.

I do warn such patients that their reproductive functions won't return to full potency on the day the antibiotic therapy is finished. It can take up to a year for the immune system to calm down and for the full benefits of antibiotic therapy to be realized. As I mentioned before, if pregnancy fails to occur right after the completion of antibiotic therapy, the chances to achieve a pregnancy are better the next month and so on all the way to the ninth or even the twelfth month. Therefore, a patient who wants to attempt IVF after antibiotic therapy is better off doing it after a few months' rest. Failure to achieve a pregnancy on clomiphene therapy leaves the patient with the option to use injectable fertility drugs without IVF or to move right on to a full IVF cycle.

In my practice, I've adopted a flexible, open-ended approach to injectable fertility drug stimulation. With every cycle I make all options available to my patients, including IVF. As the stimulation treatment proceeds, a continuous dialogue between my patient and me shapes the next action taken. If a favorable response is achieved and numerous preovulatory follicles show up on an ultrasound examination of her ovaries, she can opt for an HCG injection and then return home to try for a spontaneous conception. On the other hand, she may choose to undergo artificial insemination. Or perhaps she'll decide on a partial or complete harvest of her follicles and then combine either spontaneous intercourse or artificial insemination with partial or full in-vitro processing of oocytes. I find this type of flexible management of a cycle less stressful for the patient because she's fully aware of all the possibilities and has control of the situation.

A patient with polycystic ovarian syndrome (PCO), a chronic endocrine disorder described in Chapter 3 (see pages 63-66), is a candidate for either clomiphene or injectable hormone stimulation. PCO features elevated baseline levels of LH and insulin resistance. Some women with PCO exhibit an increased level of male hormone production by their ovaries. Typical consequences are a scanty, irregular menstruation or the absence of menstruation altogether, infertility, and diabetes. There is also a higher incidence of obesity, excess body hair, endometrial cancer, and cardiovascular disease among women with PCO.

In most PCO cases, treatment involves oral birth control pills to suppress LH and the male hormones to establish a normal menstrual cycle. At this time, treatment with clomiphene is often enough to facilitate successful ovulation. In cases where Type-II diabetes has developed, other insulin-sensitizing agents such as glucophage (metformin) and rezulin (troglitazone), followed by clomiphene, are commonly used to achieve the same result. PCO patients tend to respond more readily to injectable drugs. To avoid dangerous hyperstimulation, close monitoring is needed.

Reviewing this section on hormone therapy, you can appreciate the multiple factors to be considered in each case before the doctor and the patient, working together, can design the safest and most promising hormone therapy. Unless attention is paid to differences in individual responses to these powerful remedies and every patient is handled individually, optimum results cannot be expected.

Finally, I have to say a few words about the safety of these drugs and the long-term side effects. I mentioned the hyperstimulation syndrome, when the formation of too many follicles can create a life-threatening condition. Fortunately, this condition is becoming a rarity thanks to the now routine use of serial hormone and ultrasound examinations to monitor what's going on. However, multiple-birth pregnancies resulting from hormone stimulation are here to stay and often present health concerns.

Scientific research has shown that there's a definite increase in the incidence of benign ovarian tumors among women who have received fertility drugs during their reproductive years. Whether or not there is an increase in the number of malignant ovarian tumors among the same patient population has not yet been proven.

Infertility in itself is associated with a higher than average chance to develop ovarian cancer. Is it possible that the cancer-causing agent in the ovary at the same time renders the woman infertile? Or is it possible that fertility drugs, while indiscriminately stimulating the ovarian cells for follicular maturation, also stimulate dormant cancer cells? Future studies will be needed to shed light on these questions [14-16].

For all the reasons I've discussed above (some in very technical language to give you a better idea what you may hear from doctors), I firmly object to the common practice among physicians of handing out clomiphene prescriptions to women who complain of infertility and then, without any further testing, telling them to come back in a few months. Even worse, when a pregnancy fails to occur within a few months, doctors often steer patients directly toward IVF. That is why I so strongly recommend that infertile couples consult a reproductive endocrinologist—a doctor who is specially qualified to treat infertility—before engaging in any kind of therapy or procedure.

Artificial Insemination

Artificial insemination, the simplest form of ART, involves a doctor injecting sperm by means of a special instrument directly into the woman's reproductive system. The procedure has been practiced since ancient times and can now take several forms. The simplest one is depositing seminal fluid into the vagina or cervical canal. There is no special preparation of the seminal fluid, and the only mechanical devices used may be a syringe to deliver the sperm and a cervical cup or a vaginal sponge to keep the seminal fluid in place. The procedure can be performed without any technical help. Except for the inability of a couple to perform spontaneous intercourse, there are no other medical indications or therapeutic advantages to this procedure.

Due to the presence of potentially infectious bacteria and strong chemical agents, like prostaglandins, in untreated seminal fluid, it is not advisable to deposit whole semen higher up in the female genital tract, such as in the uterus or in the tubes. Instead sperm wash and swim up techniques are used to prepare sperm for intrauterine insemination (IUI) or intratubal insemination (ITI).

The use of IUI or ITI to overcome a low sperm count or other sperm problems is discussed below, under "MEN, artificial insemination." From the perspective of women's infertility problems, the most common condition prompting the use of IUI is hostile cervical mucus.

As I've mentioned in previous chapters, many doctors or clinics utilize IUI to overcome hostile cervical mucus without first trying to eliminate the pathogens making it hostile, so that sperm can penetrate it during normal intercourse. IUI certainly does the job more quickly, but at a high risk: any resulting pregnancy may allow the pathogens in the cervical mucus to spread throughout the woman's reproductive system, jeopardizing not only the health of the child and mother, but also the couple's future fertility. Unfortunately, there are as yet no scientific follow-up studies analyzing the number of secondary infertility situations created by IUI pregnancies. I suspect, however, that this rate is significantly high because of infections introduced by the IUI and then spread by the pregnancy itself. In my clinical experience, once a good post-coital test is documented, there are no added benefits to be realized by performing IUI or ITI (17, 18).

Nevertheless, IUI may serve as the only viable means of delivering sperm for natural fertilization in the following situations:

- when the cervical mucus remains hostile even after it's been treated for pathogens as thoroughly as possible;

- when supplementation with estrogen in a clomiphene cycle is ineffective; or

- when the cervical area is permanently damaged following an extensive cone biopsy for cervical abnormality.

It's also the mechanism by which donor sperm (sperm that are not from the woman's partner) are transferred to her uterus: a process that should also only take place after the woman's cervical mucus and reproductive system as a whole have been treated for pathogens as effectively as possible. IUI is commonly practiced in combination with clomiphene and gonadotropin stimulation (19).

ITI is a variant of artificial insemination. I am unaware of any scientific proof that this procedure provides added benefits or that any particular infertility situation legitimately calls for its use.

Once a bona fide indication for IUI is established, its timing should coincide with ovulation. In my practice, the patient is instructed to use the urine predictor kit to determine this time. When the color changes to indicate ovulation, she calls my office, and the couple comes for the procedure the following morning. Single or back-to-back inseminations can be performed in subsequent days.

First, freshly obtained sperm is washed in commercially available solutions and then centrifuged. From the resulting pellet, the most active sperms break away first into a superimposed droplet. Using sterile conditions, this small volume of most active sperm is then entirely injected into the uterus. If the timing is right and pregnancy fails to occur in three successive IUI trials, there is no point in pursuing further insemination.

In Vitro Fertilization (IVF)

IVF is a four-stage procedure:

- First, powerful drugs are used for super ovulation (forcing the formation of multiple eggs for the month).

- The eggs are removed from the ovary by minor surgery.

- The eggs are combined with sperm in a culture dish where, hopefully, fertilization takes place ("in vitro" is Latin for "in glass;" the common expression for a child produced by IVF is "test tube baby.")

- A transfer procedure sets the fertilized eggs inside the uterus where, hopefully, at least one will implant itself in the uterine lining, and a natural pregnancy will commence.

An IVF procedure features different kinds of drugs at different stages. First, birth control pills and different FSH and LH neutralizing drugs (such as lupron) are used to prepare the ovaries and to suppress the woman's own cycle. Then a powerful injectable preparation containing either pure FSH or a mixture of FSH and LH is administered until blood hormone measurements and pelvic ultrasound examinations show that the number and size of follicles in the ovary are adequate. An HCG injection helps complete the maturation of these follicles. The last group of drugs—antibiotics, steroids, estrogen, and progesterone—aims to suppress potential infections and immune reactions, and to boost the development of the uterine lining.

The odds are high that an IVF procedure won't result in a pregnancy. The technological process in itself has only been available since 1978. Because it still impresses all of us as a wondrous breakthrough in medical science, a true "modern miracle," it tends to be overrated as a means of conquering infertility. In fact, only 29.10 percent of IVF procedures were reported to be successful in 1998, the last year for which statistics are available (Fertility and Sterility, 2002,

77:18-31). This means that the average case of IVF has a 70.90 percent chance of failing.

Paradoxically (or maybe not, given our money-oriented culture), IVF also commands respect because it's so expensive. One cycle can cost anywhere from ten to fifteen thousand dollars. Many patients can't help feeling that the more something costs, the better it is in every respect, including in its chances for success. Unfortunately, no one can deny the financial interest the medical community has in promoting IVF, and this helps account for how often it is recommended.

IVF certainly deserves credit for enabling thousands of otherwise infertile women to give birth. The problem is that doctors frequently recommend it when it may not be necessary. Several of the infertility conditions they most commonly attempt to override with IVF are ones that can be corrected much more simply and inexpensively with antibiotic therapy or with hormone supplements. Among others, these conditions include sperm-antibody problems; endometriosis; dry cervical milieu; infertility following any kind of pelvic infection, provided the tubes remain intact; and the majority of so-called "unexplained" infertility cases.

In recent years, a sobering criticism of the IVF-centered mentality among Americans has been coming from the European medical community. Recent multi-center trials conducted in Europe show without question that patients with the same infertility histories as those who enrolled in this country's IVF programs could get pregnant without IVF given proper time and medication (20).

When is it clearly appropriate to consider IVF? Strictly from a medical point of view, the single infertility condition among women that justifies IVF is blocked fallopian tubes, in these cases there is simply no other way but IVF to get the egg and the sperm together for fertilization. From the male point of view, severe oligospermia can be overcome with IVF. From a practical perspective, if there's not much time to devote to therapy as a whole, IVF can allow patients and their doctors to forego months or even years of trying other treatments and procedures.

Many people who have a medical or practical need for IVF have had their natural fertility destroyed by an infection. I therefore believe it's still an essential first step for such patients to undergo antibiotic therapy to clear the reproductive system of pathogens as thoroughly as possible before the IVF is attempted. Otherwise, any resulting pregnancy will boost and spread these pathogens, greatly increasing the risk of a miscarriage or an unhealthy baby.

If a man has severe oligospermia, this condition also justifies considering IVF. Often the IVF procedure itself has to be expanded to include ICSI (intracytoplasmic sperm injection) to compensate for poor sperm motility or other sperm-related problems.

Currently most people who end up in an IVF program carry the diagnosis of unexplained infertility. As I mentioned above, my clinical experience shows that in the majority of these cases the infertility is caused by an undiagnosed infection, with or without an immune reaction and with or without a structurally damaged pelvis.

Before my first book was published and my website opened (early 1990s), oral and/or intravenous antibiotic therapy was offering this group of patients a 60 percent chance for a spontaneous pregnancy within the first nine months following therapy. Since then, the average age among my patient population has gradually increased, not only because people over the same time period have been having babies later in life, but also because more people have been coming to me after having failed with other doctors, so I'm often not the first consulting physician. Today the histories of my patients tend to be more complicated and almost all of them have gone through one or multiple IVF cycles. Even so, a recent review of my antibiotic-treated patients who came to me with the diagnosis "unexplained infertility" shows a remarkable 45 percent rate of spontaneous pregnancy following therapy. These pregnancies have occurred anytime from one month to a year following the completion of the therapy. With all the scientific advances of recent years, even the most excellent IVF programs do not produce similar pregnancy rates in that same patient group.

I have a host of other objections to the prevailing custom in our culture of over-utilizing IVF. Beyond my natural aversion to substituting anything mechanized for the natural process whenever restoration of the latter is possible, I think that IVF can impose a cruel financial burden on infertile couples. The most expensive antibiotic therapy, involving both husband and wife and given intravenously along with intrauterine washings, adds up to seven thousand dollars. Also, it's a one-time treatment course that positively impacts the couple's overall health while improving fertility. By contrast, the average cycle in an IVF program costs in excess of ten thousand dollars and can sometimes be as expensive as twenty thousand dollars. Before even starting an IVF cycle, patients need to understand that IVF is a "numbers game" and often involves two or three cycles. In the United States over an average of $58,000 is spent for every live born IVF baby [21, 22].

The cost of IVF is not only financial. For the couple undergoing IVF, it involves a complete interruption of intimate life and a roller coaster of emotional, sexual and marital problems. Also, the powerful drugs used in IVF can have long-term negative physical effects on the woman's body, particularly on her ovaries.

Finally, for generations to come, it creates unpredictable genetic and reproductive costs: assuming the parents' reproductive systems are not completely cleared of infectious agents before the IVF is attempted (which is often the case), their infant will most likely be born already contaminated with vertically transmitted pathogens.

In cases when IVF results in a successful pregnancy, the mother's system, which most likely does not perform properly due to a bacterial infection, is over-stimulated. The excess hormone supply helps suppress an immune reaction primed by this infection, and the transfer of abundant in-vitro fertilized embryos to the mother's uterus increases the odds that one will implant itself into the infected lining. An ever-growing body of medical literature shows that among IVF pregnancies there is an excess of every known pregnancy-related complication [23]. Unfortunately, not only are the pregnancies and deliveries more complicated, but also there are significant health problems in the newborns [24]. Accompanying an IVF procedure with ICSI brings about an increased number of offspring with chromosomal damage [25]. I attribute the majority of these complications encountered with IVF babies to an untreated infection, the original cause of the couple's infertility. The infection, serving as a pregnancy-preventing filter, was breached by IVF, ignoring the unsuitable reproductive environment.

I'm convinced that the full-blown effect of this type of practice will be a future explosion in the number of medical diseases, all propagated by infections. Along with this explosion will come a correspondingly reduced rate of fertility.

Immunotherapy

As you found out in Chapter 3, infections entering the body can give rise to the formation of antibodies that can negatively affect any part of a man's or woman's reproductive system. Antibodies directed against ovarian or testicular tissues can cause fast depletion of these organs. Sperm-attacking antibodies produced either within the male or female genital canal can reduce sperm motility, impede sperm transfer through the female genital canal, or prevent sperm-egg interaction during fertilization.

IUI is commonly used in an effort to overcome antibody-related infertility, but there is no proof that it actually does. In theory, IVF does so by over-stimulating the female cycle and, therefore, generating high levels of female hormones: these hormones, steroids by definition, presumably suppress the antibodies. I am not aware of any scientific evidence that supports this theory.

Medical science is currently focusing great attention on the possible role that an overworking immune system may play in cases of recurring miscarriages. Endometrial biopsies of women in this category frequently show elevated levels of natural killer cells produced by the immune system, and screening of their blood often reveals varying degrees of autoimmune reactivity to body tissues (the scientific names for some of these antibodies include antiphospholipid, anti-DNA, anti-nucleotide, anti-cardiolipine, anti-thyroid, lupus, and rheumatoid factors).

Possible therapies to reverse an autoimmune system that's run amok in these ways involve aspirin, heparin, dexamethasone, progesterone, Celexa, Folgard, Intravenous Immune Globulin (IV IgG), leukocyte immunization, and Glucophage. Whether or not these therapies work remains controversial. In a recent trial, women with a history of three or more prior miscarriages and no more then one live birth were divided randomly into two groups: one group received immunotherapy and the other, a placebo. The immunotherapy did not provide any more significant beneficial effects in preventing further miscarriages than the placebo did [26].

Surgery

Once surgery was commonly performed on the cervix for stenosis (too narrow) or incompetence (too weak), but this kind of treatment is now a thing of the past. Both of these conditions are, in most cases, related to infections, although surgical biopsies or repeated freezing can also lead to narrowing of the cervical canal. As long as menstrual flow can escape through the cervix, sperm entry is not obstructed and surgery is unnecessary.

In rare instances, severe infection can lead to complete obstruction of the cervix, in which case the menstrual flow backs into the abdominal cavity and causes severe menstrual pain. Even less common are congenital abnormalities of the cervix, such as duplication or underdevelopment. Any of these situations warrant surgical correction of the cervix.

Congenital abnormalities of the uterus requiring surgery can involve the partial or complete duplication of the uterine body as well as the cervix, or else the partial or complete absence of one side of the uterus, along with associated tubal abnormalities. For women who have experienced habitual abortions, some doctors recommend operating on the septum, a partition inside the uterus. This is a highly controversial practice. The same is true for surgeries performed to remove submucosal myomas and even, in some cases, large fibroids located on the outside of the uterus or in its wall.

In any of these controversial situations, the doctor needs to evaluate the patient's symptoms with special care and weigh those symptoms carefully against potential complications that might affect the pregnancy or delivery, before surgery is undertaken. Post-surgical adhesions that develop in the uterine lining (so-called Asherman's syndrome) are almost always due to an infection. Hysteroscopic surgical removal of these adhesions is justified in an attempt to restore fertility.

Because of the delicate structure of the fallopian tubes, surgery should always be the last resort for treating them, even in cases where an obvious anatomical abnormality exists. When surgery is done, it should involve the most sophisticated microsurgery via laparoscopy, in which surgeons, guided by visual transmissions, are able to pass miniature surgical instruments or laser beams into the abdominal cavity through thin operating tubes. No matter how carefully the tubal surgery is accomplished, it is bound to leave behind a scarred area, a potential site for a future ectopic pregnancy.

With the improvement of IVF techniques, reconstructive tubal surgeries have been largely abandoned. Lately it has been shown that the rate of IVF success for women with one or two severely damaged tubes is greater after the surgical removal of the damaged tube(s).

Surgery is still widely performed to alleviate endometriosis and to remove symptomatic or asymptomatic pelvic adhesions around the tubes and ovaries. However, wedge resection of the ovaries to treat polycystic ovaries is another outmoded practice. Some doctors report beneficial results from aspirating the follicles of women who have polycystic ovaries. Before a woman undergoes radiation treatment for any pelvic malignancy, it may be advisable to have her ovaries surgically "tucked" to remove them from the radiated field and thereby preserve their fertility.

MEN

Artificial Insemination

Other than erectile dysfunction, the most common cause of infertility among men is a low sperm count or inferior sperm quality. The latter problem could be poor motility (in common language, sperm that are "bad swimmers") or poor morphology (sperm with physical deformities).

Not uncommonly, these problems can be infection-related and can be improved or overcome entirely by antibiotic therapy. When medical therapy to improve sperm parameters doesn't succeed, the only way to improve the numerical odds is through artificial insemination (or, in cases of severe oligospermia, IVF). Simultaneously giving clomiphene or gonadotropin to the female to achieve superovulation further improves the odds.

For artificial insemination, the ejaculate is taken from the man. It is then processed to create a higher concentration of good quality sperm. The sperm is washed and centrifuged several times with commercially available solutions. The final pellet with all the washed sperm in it is allowed to stand in the bottom of a test tube with a small amount of clear nourishing fluid layered above it. The most active, healthiest sperm break away from the pellet and swim to the top, thus leaving poorly moving deformed sperm and debris in the bottom. This upper fluid is then collected and injected either into the woman's uterus or into her fallopian tubes (or, in cases of IVF, into a culture medium containing the woman's eggs).

IVF can help a man with very severe sperm problems to overcome infertility. The few available sperm are collected, washed, concentrated and finally, with extremely delicate instruments, injected into mature eggs. However, it bears repeating that this procedure bypasses one of nature's screens to prevent not only infections from being horizontally and vertically transmitted but also chromosomal abnormalities in the sperm from being passed along to offspring. Thorough testing needs to be done in advance for pathogens as well as for chromosomal abnormalities, and appropriate steps taken accordingly.

Surgery

By far the most common form of surgery performed on infertile men is the correction of a swollen or varicose vein in the scrotum (varicocele). This condition occurs when gravity in erect humans aggravates congenitally weakened veins in the scrotum. The dilated veins then effectively interfere with heat elimination from the testicles. In this situation, the heat and, probably, the backflow of some toxic substances from the kidneys can cause depressed sperm production (oligospermia), reduced motility, and/or certain structural aberrations in sperms.

Varicocele affects roughly 10 percent of all men and 40 percent of men who seek medical help for infertility. In most cases, the surgical solution for varicocele is to cut and tie the vein so there is no back flow of blood. Other approaches include using a silicone balloon to occlude the blood supply or an embolization technique to obliterate the blood vessels. For all procedures, there is a 20 percent chance of recurrence.

Surgery provides a fast answer but it isn't necessarily the best one. Many doctors push for surgery much too quickly, before they've devoted a sufficient amount of time to microbiological testing and antibiotic therapy. Genital tract infections can cause sperm abnormalities that are indistinguishable from those created by a varicocele. There are also patients with a combination of abnormalities from both an infection and a varicocele.

A varicocele results in poor sperm quality, which, in turn, means that few if any sperm are available for fertilization or for transport of infections to the female partner's internal genital tract. If infections are ignored in infertility treatment, a quick pregnancy that follows varicocele repair can have a very damaging effect on the uterus. The short and long term implications of this infection for both mother and child are discussed elsewhere in this book. On rare occasions, we have seen outright PID developing very shortly after varicocele repair.

Antibiotic therapy is always advisable as a first step in the treatment of a varicocele. Aside from cleaning the man's reproductive tract in general, antibiotic therapy may well bring the overall semen parameters to a fertile level, despite the continuing presence of his varicocele.

Another structural problem causing elevated scrotal temperature and a low sperm count is hydrocele. In this condition a large amount of fluid collects between tissue layers that then compresses the testicle. The result is an overheating that impedes sperm production and a reduction of the blood supply to the testicle. Left untreated for many years, hydrocele can even cause the testicle to atrophy. Like a varicocele, the hydrocele is corrected by cut-and-stitch occlusion surgery.

From the standpoint of fertility, there is a profound difference between congenital inguinal hernias and the inguinal hernias that can be acquired in later life. During the development of the embryo, the well-formed, intact fetal testes conduct their own descent, opening and closing the abdominal wall so that they can hang outside the body. Unilateral or bilateral undescended testes always point to some damage of the testes suffered inside the uterus, including partial or complete absence of the sperm-forming structures and/or different degrees of damage to the male hormone-producing cells. Accordingly, the affected man can have a spectrum of fertility problems, from minimal reduction in sperm count to complete sterility. There is a statistically high incidence of malignant tumors among men with undescended testes, so surgical correction or removal of those testes is always recommended.

Men with a congenitally absent vas deferens or with a vas deferens that has later been obstructed by an infection or trauma may also be advised to get surgical correction. Lately, however, this solution to the problem has been replaced more and more with a micro-aspiration technique for collecting sperms to use in IVF cycles.

Some men use a THD (testicular hypothermia device) to keep the scrotum and, therefore, the sperm at a properly cool temperature. In essence, a THD is a modified pair of jockey shorts permeated with a volatile liquid. Evaporation of this liquid cools the testes and yields comparable results to surgery. Although users and their doctors have reported unquestionable success stories, this method has never become a popular alternative to varicocele surgery because the THD is very cumbersome for long-term wearing.

Thayer, one of my early patients in the 1970s, did choose to wear a THD to overcome his varicocele, and it apparently accomplished its purpose. There were, however, problems associated with this case that make it worth discussing in a bit more detail.

When I first told Thayer about his varicocele, I recommended surgery, but he was terrified at this prospect. Instead, he wore the bulky, uncomfortable jockey shorts for three months without interruption (the minimum period advisable for the full sperm-generating process to take place). Frankly I was amazed at the positive results in his sperm count. After finding bacteria in his semen sample, I advised him to proceed with a course of antibiotic therapy and then try for a spontaneous pregnancy.

At the time, I did not know as much about the seriousness of infections as I do now, so when Thayer chose not to follow-up with antibiotic therapy, I didn't pursue the idea. Within three months, his wife Essie was pregnant. She carried the child two weeks past her due date and responded poorly to Pitocin induction, so their son, Kirk, was delivered by cesarean section.

Fortunately, Kirk was in good health. Unfortunately, his mother was not. She went into severe postpartum depression after his birth. It took over a year of prescription drugs and psychotherapy for her to recover. Meanwhile, her period showed a brownish spotting and a shortened flow.

Thayer had stopped wearing the THD as soon as the pregnancy had been confirmed; but after eight months off the device, he returned out of curiosity to have his semen sample checked. The sperm parameters were as poor as they had been when I first diagnosed his varicocele-related infertility.

A few years later, when I found out that Thayer and Essie wanted to try for another pregnancy, I sat down with them for a serious discussion about what had gone wrong the last time: something about which I was much better informed at this stage in my career. I told them it was my belief that the untreated infection found in Thayer's semen sample had been the cause of the failed labor induction, the need for the cesarean section, Essie's postpartum depression, and the adverse changes in her menstruation.

Both Thayer and Essie agreed to bacteria testing and, based on that, a lengthy therapy of Erythromycin and Doxycycline. In addition, Thayer began wearing the THD again. As time went by, I witnessed a rapid improvement in Thayer's semen quality, both in terms of the sperm parameters and the disappearance of pathogens.

I was also pleased to learn that Essie's menstruation had returned to normal. Within four months a child was conceived. On the due date, their daughter, Dana, was born through vaginal delivery. Both Dana and her brother continue to be healthy individuals. There was no postpartum depression and the menstrual periods returned without change.

Hormone Therapy

When a man's pituitary gland fails to produce a sufficient amount of FSH and LH, he develops a condition referred to as pituitary hypogonadism. The cause is either unknown (idiopathic) or a secondary problem following surgery or trauma to the pituitary gland. This deficiency results in a low sperm count (oligospermia, which can also be caused by other factors, as discussed above). Treatment consists of long-term administration of FSH and LH (via the drugs Pergonal and Repronex). A typical regimen featuring these drugs is biweekly injections of 75 unit vials for five to six months until the man's testosterone has risen to an acceptable level and the sperm count has reached a fertile range. Unless maintenance injections are given, gradual deterioration of semen quality takes place within three months. This is the only male-related reproductive problem for which hormone therapy has proven effective.

A much larger group of men with oligospermia falls into the idiopathic group. It's not uncommon for doctors to prescribe clomiphene for this condition. In my opinion, this strategy has never proven to be effective. Some authorities cite incidents in which the sperm count has risen in the months following clomiphene intake, but any connection between these two events has yet to be firmly established. Month by month an oligospermic man's sperm count can vary radically and randomly whether or not he's receiving treatment.

OTHER OPTIONS FOR COUPLES

Certain insurmountable problems may require outside help. When a woman's eggs are damaged due to age or infection, donor eggs are the only option. Through IVF, another woman's eggs are fertilized with the man's sperm. Any resulting embryos are then implanted into the uterus of the would-be mother. Anonymous donors are either young, healthy volunteers or women designated by the recipient, usually close relatives. Any potential donor is first screened according to strict state laws.

If a man is azoospermic (no sperm in his ejaculate), or has a sperm count too low for an IVF cycle, or has some genetic factor that makes his sperm unusable, donor sperm can provide an alternative. Washed donor sperm can be injected directly into the woman's uterus or fallopian tube. In cases where tubal problems exist, or any other indication for IVF is encountered, washed donor sperm can be used in an IVF cycle.

Sperm donors for clinics and sperm banks are young, healthy males who are recruited and screened according to strict state laws. Following the screening, the donor is allowed to donate at set time intervals. The samples are frozen and quarantined in liquid nitrogen for six months. At that point certain laboratory tests are repeated on the donor. If his tests are still negative for a set number of diseases, the sperm samples are released for clinical use.

Another way to help guarantee a disease-free donor is to select only a married donor in a stable relationship that has produced healthy children. During my clinic's selection process for sperm donors, the obstetric history of the donor's wife and the health histories of their children are far more reassuring than the man's entirely negative laboratory report presented to the health department.

Sometimes a treatment-resistant infectious or structural problem in the woman's reproductive system makes it impossible for her to sustain a pregnancy. In these situations, first her eggs are fertilized by the man's sperm via IVF. Any resulting embryos are then implanted in the uterus of another woman who ultimately gives birth to the baby. The would-be parent who provides the egg is called the egg donor, and the woman who undertakes the pregnancy is called the surrogate mother. Despite the facts that altruistic, informal surrogacy arrangements do occur, the majority of surrogate mothers are strangers, hired by the infertile couple, who require a preconceptional agreement that includes a payment schedule.

Inherent in the surrogacy process are numerous problems of a morally and legally ambiguous nature. The validity of the surrogate mother's consent may be debatable: she may, for example, be influenced to consent by a psychological problem. Alternatively, it's possible that the surrogacy experience itself will cause her psychological harm in the future. There is also the issue of whether or not the surrogacy set-up exploits the financial need of the surrogate mother. And there is the risk that the surrogate mother's health may be adversely affected, or she herself may cause complications, if either of the genetic parents suffers a major disease or untimely death during or after the surrogacy. Surrogacy contracts are covered by state law, so to prevent protracted litigation or injustice to anyone involved, couples that choose this route are advised to seek good legal advice.

CHAPTER 5 REFERENCES

1. Filicori M., Santoro N., Merriam G.R., Crowley Jr. WF. "Characterization of physiological pattern of episodic gonadotropin secretion throughout the human menstrual cycle. *J Clin Endocrinol Metab*, 1986; 62: 1136.
2. Urban R.J., Veldhuis J.D., Dufau M.L. "Estrogen regulates the gonadotropin-releasing hormone-stimulated secretion of biologically active luteinizing hormone." *J Clin Endocrinol Metab*, 1991; 72:660.
3. Mortola J.F., Laughlin G.A., Yen SSC. "A circadian rhythm of serum follicle-stimulating hormone secretion in women." *J Clin Endocrinol Metab*, 1992; 75: 861.
4. Liu J.H., Yen S.S.C. "Induction of midcycle gonadotropin surge by ovarian steroids in women: a critical evaluation." *J Clin Endocrinol Metab*, 1983; 57: 797.
5. Sherman B.M., Korenman S.G. "Hormonal characteristics of the human menstrual cycle throughout reproductive life." *J Clin Invest*, 1975; 55: 699.
6. Lee S.J., Lenton E.A., Sexton L., Cooke I.D. "The effect of age on the cycle patterns of plasma LH, FSH, estradiol and progesterone in women with regular menstrual cycle." *J Clin Endocrinol Metab*, 1988; 3: 851.
7. Schlecht J.A. "Clinical impact of Hyperprolactinemia." *J Clin Endocrinol Metab*, 1995; 9: 359.
8. Kredentser J.V., Hoskins C.F., Scott J.Z. "Hyperprolactinemia—a significant factor in female infertility." *Obstet Gynecol*, 1981; 139: 264.
9. Poppe K., Glinoer D., Van Steirteghem A., Tournaye H., Devroey P.., Achiettecatte J., Velkeniers B. "Thyroid dysfunction and autoimmunity in infertile women." *Thyroid*, 2002; 12: 997-1001.
10. Krassas G.E. "Thyroid disease and female reproduction." *Fertil Steril*, 2000; 74: 1063-70.
11. Strauss J.F., Steinkampf M.P. "Pituitary-ovarian interactions during follicular maturation and ovulation." *Am J Obstet Gynecol*, 1995; 172: 726-35.
12. van Zonnewald P., te Velde E.R., Koppeschaar H.P. "Low luteal phase serum progesterone levels in regularly cycling women are predictive for subtle ovulation disorders." *Gynecol Endocrinol*, 1994; 8: 169-74.
13. Gleicher N., Oleske D.M., Tor-Kaspa I., Vidali A., Karande V. "Reducing the risk of high-order multiple pregnancy after ovarian stimulation with gonadotropins." *N Eng J Med*, 2000; 343: 2-7.
14. The Eshre Capri Workshop. "Guidelines to the prevalence, diagnosis, treatment and management of infertility." In: Crosignami PG, Rubin E. eds. *Excerpts on Human Reproduction. No 4.* Oxford, England: Oxford University Press, 1996: 5-28.

15. Fauser B., Van Heusen A.M. "Manipulation of human ovarian function: physiological concepts and clinical consequences." *Endocrine Rev,* 1997; 18: 71-106.

16. The Collaborative Ovarian Cancer Group, Whittemore A.S., Harris R., Itnyre J. "Characteristics relating to ovarian cancer risk: collaborative analysis of 12 US case-control studies." II. "Invasive epithelial ovarian cancers in white women." *Am J Epidemiol,* 1992; 136: 1184-203.

17. Stuart J.A. "Stimulated intra-uterine insemination is not a natural choice for the treatment of unexplained subfertility: Should the guidelines be changed?" *Hum Reprod,* 2003; 18: 903-907.

18. Snick H. "Is the benefit of IUI really evidence-based?" *Hum Reprod,* 2002; 17: 3003-3004.

19. Guzik D.S., Carson S.A., Coutifaris C. "Efficacy of superovulation and intrauterine insemination in the treatment of infertility." *N Eng J Med,* 1999; 340: 177-183.

20. Vogin G.D. "Assisted reproduction should be postponed for healthy women." In ESHRE Annual Meeting July 3, 2002.

21. Neumann P., Soheyla D. Gharib D.. Weinstein M.C. "The cost of a successful delivery with in vitro fertilization." *New Eng J Med,* 1994; 331: 239-243.

22. Gerseau L., Henderson J., Davis L.J., et al. "Economic implications of assisted reproductive techniques: a systemic review." *Hum Reprod,* 2002; 17: 3090-3109

23. Bergh T., Ericson A., Hillensjo T., Nygren K.G., Wennerholm U.B. "Deliveries and children born after in vitro fertilization in Sweden 1982-95: a retrospective cohort study." *Lancet,* 1999; 354: 1579-1585.

24. Shieve L.A., Meikle S.F., Ferre C., Peterson H.B., Jeng G., Wilcox L.S. "Low and very low birth weight in infants conceived with the use of assisted reproductive technology." *New Eng J Med,* 2002; 346:731-737.

25. Wennerholm U.B., Bergh C., Hamberger L., et al. "Incidence of congenital malformations in children born after ICSI." *Hum Reprod,* 2000; 15: 944-948.

26. Scott JR. "Immunotherapy for recurring miscarriage (Cochrane Review)." In: *The Cochrane Library,* Issue 2, 2003. Oxford, Eng.

CHAPTER 6

THE FERTILE FUTURE

We are at our best when we give the doctor
who resides within each patient a chance to go to work.
—Dr. Albert Schweitzer

It is possible to fail in many ways...
while to succeed is possible only in one way.
—Aristotle

People outside the medical profession tend to trust in the efficiency of infertility treatment in general. After all, isn't it one of the more "advanced" sciences, associated with the impressive headlines we see so often these days about genetic engineering and cloning? Isn't it related to physiology, biology, and technology so complex and specialized that they go way beyond the bounds of "ordinary" knowledge? What right does the non-medical person have to question it?

Because of this attitude, actual and prospective patients are inclined to trust infertility experts more or less blindly. This is especially true in the case of ART procedures, which are impressive in their own right simply because of the sophisticated gadgetry involved.

Understandably, infertile people want desperately to believe in any potential solution to their problem and, as a result, can easily find themselves entering into this kind of unquestioning trust. However, it is a dangerous state of mind and very close to what psychologists call denial: "I don't want to give due consideration to the uncertainties—I don't want to face the possibility of complications or failure." In fact, if you're a prospective parent who faces reliance on infertility treatment, it is essential that you give deep personal consideration to these issues, not only for the benefit of yourself, your relationship with your partner, and any child you may have, but also for the benefit of humanity.

The science of infertility treatment is still very new and comparatively untested, and ART is the youngest and most unproven sector within it. Many couples who put all their hopes into IVF, for example, don't realize or forget that the first successful IVF took place less than three decades ago. It remains a risky new strategy, and we have no firm basis yet for determining what the full spectrum of long-range consequences may be for the parent or the child [1-3].

I have already discussed some of the potentially negative consequences of IVF treatment, given certain conditions. You can now appreciate that if a woman with a neglected or insufficiently treated infection in her lower reproductive tract conceives through IVF, the subsequent pregnancy may contaminate her upper reproductive tract and render her permanently infertile and unhealthy. You're also now aware that the same woman, because of her pregnancy-escalated infection, may give birth to an unusually sickly child who will pass along a higher-than-usual number of major illnesses to future generations. These post-IVF outcomes may be far more likely—or problematic—than we're yet able to verify, and there may well be a host of other worrisome outcomes or scenarios that we've so far not even imagined.

The future of the young, rapidly growing science of infertility treatment is bound to bring all sorts of new developments and realizations: some encouraging, others troubling. As a would-be parent heading into this bold new world, what questions do you need to address, beginning right now, that relate to how the coming years will turn out for you and your family? As human beings, what can all of us expect to happen in the society of tomorrow, and how can we help to make sure it's as positive as possible for everyone?

In this chapter we'll look more closely at these questions, starting with the personal ones and moving on to the more general ones. In addressing each question, I'll emphasize the most important points to keep in mind, based not only on all the reading you have done so far about my past and present clinical experience, but also on my research into likely future developments.

WHAT FACTORS DO I NEED TO CONSIDER IN PLANNING A FAMILY?

Bringing a child into the world—which begins when you're selecting a mate and ends when your son or daughter has reached a reasonably self-sufficient maturity—is not an experience that can be isolated from the rest of your life. It is a process that influences, and is affected by, every other aspect of your existence: your health, your relationships, your financial status, your work, your play, your dreams and ambitions. You need to examine each aspect carefully in light of the others, to make sure that everything fits together in a practical pattern. This requires taking stock of what you know, doing research about what you don't know, and clarifying your goals in each area to the point where you have a better sense of the future activities, resources, and timeframes that they may require.

As you engage in this multidimensional life-planning, you may come to realize that various factors are in conflict with one another. For example, you may have career aspirations that would require not having children for at least five years. However, your state of reproductive health, or your partner's, may indicate that you're taking an enormous risk to wait that long to reproduce. In this case, you may want to readjust your career objectives and/or your plans for a family.

On the other hand, all the media scare stories may well have convinced you that a "normal" woman's fertility begins diminishing radically in her thirties, so that it is inherently risky for her to postpone having a child until her late thirties or early forties. In fact, women whose reproductive systems are healthy—undamaged by vertically or horizontally acquired pathogens—can reproduce quite readily well into their fourth decade without medical assistance. As for a man, there is a slight age-related decline in male sperm production during a man's mid-forties, but, barring pathogenic infection, his sperm are likely to remain fertile even into his seventh decade.

Infertility patients frequently ask me why so many promiscuous people, presumably at high-risk for infertility-causing infections, have so many children, quite a few unplanned or even unwanted. The answer to this question is based on the complicated interplay between the age of the human host, the pathogens, and the ability of the host's immune system to handle these pathogens. Despite irresponsible sexual practices during the teenage years, reproduction is still possible while the host is young even with the presence of some pathogens in the reproductive canal. A young person's immune system can handle infections more readily than an older person's immune system. However, if the same bacterial infection is left unattended for years, it will partially or completely shut down the reproductive process.

Young couples who share infectious bacteria often have pregnancies that go all the way to a live birth. Nevertheless, the infection is present in the delivered newborn. Meanwhile, the course of pregnancy itself has spread the infection within the woman's female reproductive canal so there is a good chance that miscarriage or secondary infertility will ensue.

Focusing strictly on health issues, we need to remember that our reproductive system's well-being is intimately connected with our physical health in general. It is also tied, somewhat more loosely, to the reproductive and physical health of our parents, our partner, our partner's parents, and so on. As you now know, this is because similar pathogens, acquired either vertically or horizontally, can cause infertility-related difficulties as well as a host of other major diseases. Therefore, problems of one kind tend to reflect actual or potential problems of the other kind.

If you are now looking for a spouse or partner with whom you want to have a child, or if you find yourself doing so in the future, you are probably going to look at each potential mate through different eyes from the first date on, based on what you've read in this book. You can easily find ways to channel casual conversations so that you can find out more about the medical and reproductive history of this person and his or her family. Better still, you and this person may quickly reach a level of mutual confidence and understanding so that you can talk about the matter more directly. Whatever the case, when the two of you are finally ready to conceive a child, I am sure you will be more prepared to invest time, energy, and money in fertility testing and, if indicated, fertility-related treatments.

If at all possible, you and your mate—now or in the future—would be wise to investigate these health matters well before you try to conceive a child, so that you have an ample amount of time and opportunity to treat any infections that may be present in your reproductive systems. However, even if you've already conceived, this investigative effort can result in better-targeted health care, a greatly reduced risk of complications throughout the pregnancy, and a much healthier child. If medical conditions prevent you from having your own child, you need to scrutinize medical and family histories of sperm and egg donors as thoroughly as you can—again, something I am confident you can appreciate based on what you have read here.

Assuming you're either seeking to overcome infertility now, or planning in advance to know more about your potential fertility, your mission is to use the questionnaires in the next chapter as a framework for collecting as much information as possible about all relevant medical and reproductive health histories affecting you and your partner. Ideally, the people you want to include in this survey (and involve in its collection) are:

- you and your partner;

- all your siblings and your partner's siblings;

- your parents and your partner's parents;

- your grandparents and your partner's grandparents;

- all your former sexual partners and those of your partner.

The next step is to consult with a reproductive endocrinologist and arrange for testing. Although this process sounds fairly simple and straightforward, you may encounter difficulties in finding a physician who is knowledgeable about, or sympathetic to, antibiotic therapy or a laboratory that is competent to facilitate the required testing. In these circumstances in particular, you need to be a persistent advocate for yourself. After all, people in the medical profession are not perfect. As in every other area of life, a certain amount of rigidity, ignorance, impersonality, and cynicism prevails.

The information you've collected with the help of the questionnaires will provide very useful background material for this consultation. A high score on the questionnaires will also provide good motivation, but to be on the safe side, you should take action right away whatever your score may be. The effect of bacterial contamination on a woman's reproductive canal and on a man's semen quality is cumulative, so each passing year can significantly add to the problem. Because of the value of early detection, I recommend bacterial testing not only as soon as possible before attempting a pregnancy, but also as a matter of routine prior to getting married and, on an individual basis, whenever any genital-tract discomfort or problem is noted, or anytime one engages in intercourse with a new partner.

Above all, I urge every individual and couple seeking treatment for infertility to go through bacterial testing and, if warranted, antibiotic treatment before undertaking any ART. I also advise them to explore all the issues involving ART before they make their decision, including the possibility of giving birth to an unhealthy child.

As I mentioned earlier in this book, the majority of ART procedures are currently performed for infertility conditions labeled "of unknown causes." I'm convinced that a significant number of these cases are caused by an undiagnosed infection or a combination of this infection and an adverse immune-system reaction to it. If you ignore the infectious component to the infertility and override it with an ART procedure, complications are inevitable, including, I believe, the proliferation of major medical diseases.

Some infertility doctors acknowledge a correlation in recent years between the increasing number of ART procedures that are performed and the surge in major medical diseases. However, they don't necessarily appreciate that it is the same infectious cause behind both phenomena. Also, many doctors still leave almost all reproductive decisions entirely up to their patient without informing them properly about the various ramifications of each possibility. Dr. Norman Gleicher of the Center for Human Reproduction in New York cautions against both forms of inattention. In a recent article in Fertility and Sterility magazine, he warned, "In overcoming...blocks toward successful reproduction [with ART], we are opening the floodgates toward higher and earlier disease prevalence in future" [4].

Other guidelines for maintaining sound medical and reproductive health are to practice good hygiene, thereby reducing the bacterial load, and to avoid drug or alcohol abuse. From the standpoint of physical health, there is a definite premium on remaining a virgin or abstaining as much as possible from sex until marriage. Rape is an even more serious crime when you consider the possibility that the victim's reproductive system can be contaminated by the perpetrator's seminal fluid.

Assuming you choose to lead an active sex life, you should always use a condom during intercourse until you are ready to conceive (at which time you should be sure that you and your partner have infection-free reproductive systems before stopping condom use). Relying on a condom rather than some other form of birth control is the only way to prevent damaging pathogens from being transmitted horizontally from one partner to the other, and this is assuming that the condom is used correctly.

WHAT CAN I DO TO HELP SAFEGUARD MY CHILD'S FERTILITY IN THE FUTURE?

You can begin by making sure your child is brought to birth in the healthiest possible reproductive system: one that is not likely to transmit pathogens to his or her body. I also advise having your child tested for pathogens in the reproductive system in late puberty (age 16-18). It should follow a frank discussion on sexuality and reproductive hygiene, so that the need for testing is clear.

If you think that your child is on the brink of engaging in sexual intercourse, arrange for expeditious testing: It's better to do it while your child is still virginal, before a pre-existing infection is exacerbated by sex or before a partner transmits a new infection. All other factors aside, testing can be appropriate for any boy who masturbates or for a girl whose sexual development is complete.

Some special circumstances also warrant testing. It is advisable if you have a daughter who starts complaining about early vaginal or bladder irritations before becoming sexual active. Another situation that calls for testing is when pre-pubertal girls rapidly develop ovarian cysts immediately following menarche: this scenario suggests the presence of a vertically acquired infection and the ascent of bacteria through the menstrual flow. Emergencies that beg for immediate testing include severe dysmenorrhea, irregular menstruation, and a menstrual period that was normal but subsequently slid into oligomenorrhea or amenorrhea.

When talking about sex and reproduction to children who are old enough to understand what bacteria are, you should mention the possibility that harmful bacteria can be transmitted horizontally during intercourse, but do so in a calm, objective way that does not cause inappropriate alarm. Your purpose is not to make your child fear sex or, in a gesture of denial or self-defense, question your motives and, therefore, the truth of what you're saying. Instead, you want to provide more information to help your child make the most sensible possible decision about how to behave sexually. With or without your explicit recommendation attached, this information will make it easier for your child to consider either abstaining from premarital sex or engaging in it more moderately and always using a condom.

WHAT ABOUT THE PREVAILING WISDOM THAT TOO MUCH INTAKE OF ANTIBIOTICS CAN RESULT IN THE DEVELOPMENT OF STRONGER, MORE RESISTANT STRAINS OF BACTERIA?

When antibiotics first began appearing for widespread public use after World War II, they seemed to most laypeople like a magic bullet that could be used to destroy almost any illness. In the decades since then, there's no question that antibiotics have often been over-prescribed by doctors and overused by patients. This kind of abuse can, indeed, build up resistant bacterial strains from the very pathogens they were meant to kill, thus gradually reducing the effectiveness of antibiotics for the person who overuses them.

In today's world, partly in reaction to the extravagant praise antibiotics previously received, the pendulum is swinging a bit too far in the other direction, with more public concern about using antibiotics than most situations warrant. In fact, medical science has proven the singular effectiveness of long-term antibiotic use in treating a number of complicated illnesses. Chronic prostatitis, for example, sometimes calls for antibiotic therapy lasting anywhere from six months to years in duration, using varying regimens. Similarly, chronic infections in elderly patients, AIDS sufferers, and cancer patients are commonly managed with lengthy antibiotic regimens. As long as the use of antibiotics is justified by the problem, tailored to treat the specific pathogens involved, and well-monitored by the physician, the risks are minimal and worth taking.

Unfortunately, antibiotic therapy sometimes fails to clear up an infection due to the presence of bacteria that already exhibit resistance to multiple kinds of drugs. In such a case, more antibiotic therapy, perhaps of a different kind, is warranted. It is simply not medically advisable for doctors to follow a routine policy of giving patients two weeks of Doxicycline therapy at the beginning of an infertility workup and then reassuring them—without proof—that any possible infections have been eradicated.

What is the alternative to using antibiotics to restore good reproductive health? If you have a pathogenic infection and don't use antibiotics—the only means of controlling or eradicating an infection—the alternative could be a miscarriage, a complicated pregnancy, a cesarean section, a stillbirth, or an unhealthy child as well as the propagation of reproductive and medical health problems in coming generations. Hormone treatments and ART techniques carry even greater health risks than antibiotics do, and many times antibiotic therapy can altogether eliminate the need for both.

Aside from the danger that extensive reliance on antibiotics may help create resistant pathogens (and the type of therapy I advise is not in itself extensive), antibiotic use carries with it the possibility of only minor adverse side effects for a small percentage of patients. These side effects include overgrowing yeast infections (with ampicillin); occasional diarrhea, allergic skin rashes, fatigue, or headaches (with clindamycin); and local irritation at the administration site (with doxicycline, Zithromax). By using intrauterine washing on their female patients, doctors can avoid the systemic side effects of toxic drugs like gentamicin on hearing, balance nerves, the liver, and the kidney, while at the same time achieving much higher and more efficient drug concentrations within the uterus. For male patients suffering from severe prostatitis, I have had success administering similar antibiotics by directly injecting them into the prostate gland transrectally with sonographic guidance. The side effects in such a situation are negligible: possible short-term local discomfort and transient hematuria (blood in the urine) or hemospermia (blood in the seminal fluid).

WHAT IS SCIENCE LIKELY TO FIND OUT IN THE NEAR FUTURE ABOUT INFERTILITY AND RELATED MATTERS?

First of all, the trend of the past ten years indicates that through scientific research we will discover more and more proof that infertility and other major diseases—even beyond the ones I've discussed in this book and list in the questionnaires—are caused by vertically or horizontally transmitted pathogens. While scientists have given most of their attention to the role of genetics in passing along physical and mental illnesses and pre-conditions, I believe this focus will shift more toward the role of bacteria, parasites, and other microbes in passing on diseases as well as their role as the prime cause of gene alteration.

Along with this shift in perspective will come the realization that some diseases now thought to be genetic in origin are, in fact, carried down through a generational line by pathogens that the fetus picks up in the uterus. Strictly as a matter of conjecture, I think it's possible that the list might include such currently baffling illnesses as Alzheimer's disease, Parkinson's disease, Lou Gehrig's disease (amyotrophic lateral sclerosis), autism, multiple sclerosis, and schizophrenia. A number of congenital abnormalities may also be connected to intrauterine infections, most notably heart defects, spina bifida, omphalocele, and a number of chromosomal defects including Down's syndrome. I further believe that the known association between periodontal disease and the risk of stroke or heart attack is due to the same abnormal bacteria affecting two different parts of the body.

Assuming we can identify the source of these exceptionally troublesome illnesses, our capacity to treat and even overcome them becomes infinitely greater. Another beneficiary will be research and therapy associated with any other medical problem transmitted in the same manner, including infertility.

Science is also likely to produce more evidence verifying the horizontal transmission of disease-causing pathogens between sexual partners: the same pathogens that can be transmitted vertically and possibly other kinds as well. Because of this verification, the list of sexually transmitted diseases (STDs) is almost certain to expand beyond the narrow group of maladies now recognized.

I also believe that medical science will be compelled to admit in the near future that the branches of obstetrics (especially high-risk obstetrics) and gynecology emerged out of the necessity to deal with conditions caused by vertically and horizontally transmitted infections in otherwise perfectly functioning female reproductive tracts. The same could be said about the highly specialized branch of reproductive endocrinology. Meanwhile, in other branches of medicine that treat heart disease, high blood pressure, kidney ailments, kidney stones, ulcerative diseases, and diabetes, antibiotic therapy will assume an even larger role.

As a corollary to all these developments, solid scientific data will emerge to confirm that, in any society, the number of major illnesses like heart disease, cancer, and the others I've suggested is directly proportionate to the number of infertility cases, complicated pregnancies, and one-child families. What's more, the data will show that the extent of major illnesses among adults is closely related to the extent of physical, mental, and emotional health problems among young children. I suspect, and hope future research will confirm, that the state of our microenvironment, the uterine cavity, influences our emotional maturation and the development of our sexual orientation.

In addition, I think research will show that emotional troubles currently labeled as PMS-related can be solidly associated with a vertically or horizontally contaminated pelvis. More evidence will also emerge that the incidence rate of marital trouble or divorce is directly tied to such infection-caused problems as bad pregnancies, unhealthy children, and the female partner's mood problems due to hormone imbalances. And science will confirm that sophisticated ART procedures, by allowing babies to develop in infected environments, tend to generate a new type of human being with clustered medical problems. In the decades to come, the medical treatment of such individuals will unfortunately lead to larger and larger health care costs. I hope that it will eventually become common knowledge that babies conceived after their parents had intravenous antibiotic therapy have very little trouble with childhood diseases, including ear infections, tonsil problems, allergies, asthma, behavior problems, and/or attention deficit disorder.

All this research I mention will inevitably reveal that certain segments of the human population are more troubled by horizontally or vertically transmitted infections than others, due to their social, economic, political, and cultural history and the impact it has had on their prevailing sexual activity and hygiene. In China, for example, statistics over the past century have shown a marked increase in infertility problems as sexual mores have become more and more liberalized. The infertility rate almost doubled from 3 percent to 5.1 percent in the last generation. During the same time period, medical scientists observed a negative change in the sperm quality among Chinese men, and IVF clinics first opened in China [5-7].

Another situation worth monitoring is the migration of people from a region where the prevalence of a certain disease is low to a region where its prevalence is high. Southeast Asians, for example, have a low prevalence of coronary artery disease compared to people who live in Europe, Australia and the US. I suspect that Southeast Asians migrating to Europe, Australia, or the U.S. acquire horizontal infections that greatly increase their risk of getting coronary artery disease. It will take careful study of two or more generations of transplanted populations before we can know for sure about such matters [8-13].

For somewhat different reasons, I'm forced to conclude that my native country, Hungary, is a highly contaminated society. Situated in the center of Europe, at the crossroads of every major population movement in that part of the world, Hungary has suffered through an average of two major wars per century for the past 600 years. It now has an exceedingly high rate not only of ulcers, heart disease, cancer, and diabetes, but also of reproductive problems. In fact, it has a negative birth rate, meaning an unusually high incidence of no-child or one-child families [14-18].

In my own practice, I have witnessed the sad heritage of Hungary's troubled socio-economic past in the lab results of Hungarian immigrant patients referred to me because I speak their native language. Almost across the board, these results have shown a heavy concentration of harmful bacteria, and it is the exception to treat one Hungarian patient whose history reveals an undisturbed record of reproductive performance.

In the United States, we're beginning to see that a similar pattern exists among minority groups with a history of oppression, poverty, and different sexual practices. For example, statistics show that African Americans suffer from a higher incidence of sexually transmitted diseases, including AIDS [19]. African American women have a higher incidence of bacterial vaginosis [20]. At the same time the ethnic group as a whole exhibits higher rates of diabetes, heart disease, cancer, premature births, abnormal pregnancies, and children afflicted with more numerous illnesses than the national average [21-35]. The following axiom is true for every ethnic group: The presence of major medical diseases adversely affects the course of pregnancies, and high-risk conditions can be expected [36-37].

Although we can almost certainly count on science to identify specific population groups as high risk for bacterial contamination, we can't be as sure that the news will be received objectively and handled compassionately. We simply have to hope that this kind of legacy will be acknowledged as a human problem that needs to be addressed humanely for everyone's benefit.

Finally, I think that the current, narrow, discrete definition of pelvic inflammatory disease (PID) will be expanded to cover a spectrum of symptoms affecting all parts of the female genital canal— from the vagina, where bacteria can enter, to the ovaries, where infections can cause hormone abnormalities. In other words, what I now know to be true from my own clinical experience will become universally accepted in the field of infertility: a mild contamination can cause a functional disturbance at any level of the reproductive tract, and this disturbance in itself can lead to infertility on a functional basis.

Specifically, an abnormal course of pregnancy, a premature delivery, a case of toxemia, or the loss of pregnancy in any trimester will be defined as the result of one or more types of PID. Individual types will most likely be labeled according to the most prominently affected area: for example, cervical (a poor post-coital test), endometrial (luteal phase defect), tubal (blocked tube), ovarian (PCO, PMS, luteal phase defect, rising FSH), or the combination of any of the above along with a failure to reproduce.

WHAT DO YOU THINK THE FUTURE HOLDS REGARDING CLONING OR GENETIC ENGINEERING?

Broadly defined, cloning is the artificial reproduction of a single individual using his or her genetic material, so that theoretically an exact duplicate is created. Genetic engineering (or eugenics) is the artificial manipulation of an embryo's or fetus's genetic material to serve different purposes, such as the elimination of diseases and abnormal conditions or, more controversially, the selection of gender or desired attributes (often dubbed in the media as the production of "designer babies").

Both of these fields are still too young and experimental to be predictable in any specific way. Undoubtedly they represent a tide of scientific inquiry that will be carried into the future, one way or the other, regardless of individual or social feelings or beliefs. Throughout human history, new technological developments have almost always been successful at eventually overcoming opposition.

The successful cloning experiment that led to the birth of the sheep Dolly in 1997 immediately raised many ethical and scientific policy questions. Citing moral reasons, many argue against interfering with the natural development of embryos in any way. However, others maintain that such "interference" is justified, given the benefits to be gained. Stem cell research, for example, can help in treating and curing diseases, and the possibility of producing live offspring by cloning carries potential applications in animal husbandry, biotechnology, transgenic and pharmaceutical production, biomedical research, and the preservation of endangered species [38, 39]. As a direct result of genetic research, science is now able to produce antibodies in plants [40], and a host of promising areas are opening up for gene therapy, including the treatment of hemophilia and cardiovascular diseases (more specifically, therapeutic angiogenesis) [41].

I personally support research into eugenics but have serious concerns about human cloning or the genetic engineering associated with creating "designer babies." I think the latter technologies are inherently ill conceived because they tamper too much with nature's own far more ingenious methods of perpetuating life and preserving species. These technologies are also in danger of developing too fast, before we know enough about the microbiology of reproduction to appreciate what they'll actually be doing to the individuals involved, to society in general, and to the future of the human race.

Although it is not openly admitted, eugenics is already broadly practiced in most infertility clinics. In selecting sperm or egg donors for a recipient, most clinics (including mine) try to find the most sought after physical and intellectual attributes. When doing selected abortions on patients with triplets or a higher number of multiple births, most clinics (including mine) always remove the one(s) with the smallest amniotic sack. With refinements in ART technologies, it is possible to identify (and therefore retain) disease free embryos by pre-conceptional genetic testing. And finally, in an ART setting, it is always the healthiest looking embryo that is transferred into the uterus.

In a manner of speaking, I think antibiotic therapy is the most successful "eugenic experiment" in modern reproductive medicine. The overall superiority of the children born after intravenous antibiotic therapy is so impressive that I expect the near future to include pre-conception management of family planning, extensive bacterial testing and a liberal use of antibiotics. As I mentioned above, I expect studies to show that pre-conceptional antibiotic therapy offers the best chance of reducing the now escalating rate of childhood diseases, including asthma, allergies, chronic colds, ear infections, tonsillitis, chronic bronchitis, and ADD. And I am convinced that follow-up studies will document a dramatic drop in the prevalence of major medical diseases such as high blood pressure, heart disease, and diabetes among the offspring conceived after proper antibiotic therapy. The dollar amount that could be saved with this type of preventive management is simply mind-boggling. Just for diabetes, the yearly health-care expenditure in the U.S. is over one hundred billion dollars, and we even spend eleven billion dollars annually taking care of asthma [42, 43].

Based on these findings, I expect major health policy changes, including a widespread campaign for education in these matters and later, most likely, legal enforcement of sound health practices like testing for pathogens. Simultaneously, I see a significant curtailment and regulation of ART activities. It may then take one or two generations to appreciate just how much the number of significant medical diseases drops.

WILL SCIENCE PROVE THAT ONE KIND OF DIET FOR THE MOTHER-TO-BE IS MORE BENEFICIAL THAN ANOTHER FOR THE FUTURE HEALTH OF THE CHILD?

Some scientists, among them Dr. David Barker, head of the Medical Research Council Environmental Epidemiology Unit at the University of Southampton in England, believe that nutritional deficiencies or imbalances during gestation may have an adverse effect on an individual's long-term health. Barker himself contends that prenatal dietary factors possibly contribute to adult heart disease, diabetes, and many of the other illnesses I associate with prenatal bacterial infection. Currently his laboratory and others, including American laboratories funded by the National Institute of Health, are investigating not only whether this thesis is true, but also whether there is a certain kind of diet that is optimal for ensuring that a fetus develops into the healthiest possible adult [44].

In my professional opinion, there is no strong connection between prenatal diet (unless some sort of extreme diet is involved) and the child's future susceptibility to major illnesses. The only exception would be if the mother ingests large amounts of drugs, alcohol, or nicotine during pregnancy, in which case the infant's overall health might be severely compromised. Furthermore, I think the average diet of an expectant mother in the United States offers no risk of creating a significant deficiency in vitamins, minerals, carbohydrates, fats, or proteins for the developing fetus.

An extremely small diet during pregnancy can result in serious long-term consequences. For example, Dutch women bearing children during the German blockade of Holland in 1944 were living on starvation rations of only 400 calories per day [45, 46]. They then gave birth to tiny babies. Despite the fact that these babies soon caught up in size and weight, they later had a much higher incidence of obesity, heart disease, diabetes, and high blood pressure, and they themselves eventually gave birth to small babies.

I believe the Dutch women in 1944 gave birth to smaller-than-average children because their meager diet compromised not only their own nourishment, but that of their babies as well. At the same time, their weakened immune systems allowed their uterine environments to become contaminated with bacteria. These pathogens were then transferred to the second generation, which also produced smaller-than-average babies. It may take another generation before the contamination dilutes itself and the reduction in infant birth weight falls below statistical significance [47-55]. I observed a similar phenomenon in the reproductive performance of daughters of DES-exposed women. The bacteria that the daughters acquired vertically perpetuated the tendency toward reproductive failure [56].

The most significant factors affecting the nourishment of the fetus are the size of the placenta and the diameter of the blood vessels developing between the uterus and the placental vessels that deliver the actual nutrients to the baby. The undisturbed development of this system depends on the purity of the uterus: in other words, its freedom from pathogenic contamination. Only a clean uterus can receive the embryo properly and create an effective system of feeding it.

Obesity, the opposite of malnutrition, is one of the most significant concerns of nutritional medicine in the United States today, and I believe there's a connection between bacterial infection in the pregnant mother and obesity in the resulting child. In 1960, overweight children represented 5 percent of the pre-puberty population. Today this number is 11 percent [57]. A person who has been overweight since infancy is altogether different physically and physiologically from a person who was of normal weight as a child and later, as an adult, gained excess weight from habitual overeating. Even if aggressive dietary measures reduce an overweight child's body to the ideal muscle/fat proportion, the person with lifetime weight problems does not become the same person as the individual who had normal ratios ever since birth. The former individual will still have a higher incidence of lifetime heart disease, elevated blood pressure, and/or diabetic complications. Aggressive weight-loss and strict dietary control will only marginally affect the risk [58]. Also, I've learned from my own clinical experience that the individual who is obese starting in childhood often experiences pregnancies characterized by miscarriages, premature or late deliveries, and an increased chance of preeclampsia most likely caused by bacterial contamination within the genital canal. With aggressive antibiotic therapy, these reproductive complications can be avoided in subsequent pregnancies. The presence of an infection would also help explain the increase in the number of birth defects among the children of women who were obese before and during the pregnancy [59-70]. I therefore tend to believe that the cause of obesity in a certain percentage of obese people is an anaerobic bacterial infection, probably acting on the liver, which affects their ability to metabolize fat: a condition called steatohepatitis. At the same time, such bacteria can also cause reproductive difficulties and other organ damage including heart disease, high blood pressure, diabetes, and reproductive difficulties [71]. In such a case, dietary measures would only marginally reduce the risk of these major health problems. Similarly, overeating in adulthood by an individual whose childhood and adolescent weights were normal only marginally increases his or her risk of these problems [72].

IS SCIENCE LIKELY TO UNCOVER MORE LINKS BETWEEN A PERSON'S MENTAL OR EMOTIONAL STATE OF BEING AND THE ABILITY TO CONCEIVE OR BEAR A CHILD?

Psychoneurobiology—or, as it is more commonly known, the study of mind-body connections—is a rapidly growing field, so there is little doubt that such links will be explored. However, the field is yet too young and uncharted for me to predict with any confidence what discoveries may lay ahead.

Certainly there can be a strong causal connection between general mental or emotional stress and infertility. Severe stress can lead a man to experience temporary, psychologically driven impotence. It can also cause a woman to cease ovulating and menstruating. The reason is that the brain controls the pituitary gland, which manufactures hormones that help trigger ovulation and subsequent menstruation. In a more indirect way, stress experienced by either partner can result in fewer acts of intercourse simply because the mood isn't right.

These situations, however, are not as frequent or as harmful in the long-term as popular opinion would have us believe. Even more rare is the mind-over-matter state known as pseudo-pregnancy or "hysterical" pregnancy. A woman experiencing this state is one who becomes so mentally and emotionally obsessed with having a child that she goes through a psychologically-triggered cessation of her period, retention of air and gas in her stomach, and dilation of her bowel. The condition can go on for several months, as the woman eats more and gains weight.

All in all, what we have is an assortment of intriguing facts relating to the link between mental or emotional factors and physical infertility. So far, however, we haven't established any major patterns among these facts or any hard evidence that suggests that a particular kind of mind-body therapy will assist a couple to overcome infertility.

Speaking more broadly about the origin of mental and emotional problems, I do think scientists will discover that many of these conditions stem from the unfavorable state of our first microenvironment, the uterine cavity, due in most cases to bacterial infections. The nine months we spend in that milieu have far more significant effects on our overall well-being than the next eight or so decades of life outside the uterus. The cleaner it is, the more likely the chromosomes we inherit from our parents will develop to their best potential. A contaminated uterine cavity not only affects our physical and reproductive development, but also the maturation of our nervous system. The list of possible resulting afflictions may well include depression, attention-deficit disorder, hyperactivity, one or more learning disorders, bipolar disorder, and obsessive-compulsive disorder as well as more nebulous problems like immaturity or ill-temperament. The incidence of all these conditions has risen steeply in recent years, and I believe the background cause is intrauterine bacterial infections during pregnancy [73, 74].

WHAT LIES IN THE FUTURE FOR INFERTILITY TREATMENT?

First and foremost, I believe that a much higher premium will be put on prevention. Policymakers may also start tackling vertically acquired infections as a major public health issue, possibly even mandating premarital testing for bacteria as part of the qualifications for a marriage license and requiring treatment of newly recognized infections. The likelihood of such actions will be enhanced once society at large begins to realize how extensively the vertically and horizontally transmitted infections undermine human health and drive up health care costs. Also, doctors will be more educated to recognize and respond to the following key danger signals indicating that a person was born with a vertically acquired bacterial infection that may be causing his/her infertility.

An individual is more likely to have been born with an infection if he or she is the product of a pregnancy complicated by:

- prematurity or post-dated delivery;

- early rupture of the amniotic membranes;

- an infection of the uterus during pregnancy;

- preeclampsia or toxemia;

- low birth weight or retarded growth, especially in connection with an inflamed placenta;

- post-partum infection, especially endometritis;

- being the only child for no apparent reason, especially when the mother experienced an infection after the birth; and

- conception after a miscarriage, with no antibiotic treatment in the interim.

Antibiotic therapy should begin to play a much more significant role in initial, pre-conception treatment of infertile individuals and couples, who now tend to immediately opt for fertility drugs and insemination at the slightest suspicion of infertility. Treatment will be customized to fit the results provided by highly specialized microbiology laboratories that play an integral role in the functioning of any competent fertility clinic. With more precise diagnoses available, the number of cases labeled "unknown cause" will dwindle. And I'm convinced that any professional dealing with reproduction will have to receive a full training in microbiology in order to do his or her job properly.

In the future, doctors will also be much more inclined to administer antibiotics during a pregnancy to avoid complications and to ensure that the resulting baby is as healthy as possible. The functional role of a fertility expert will not end at the time of conception but rather at the time of delivery. Pregnancies will be managed with a series of microbial tests and, when appropriate, antibiotic treatment to prevent or manage complications during the pregnancy. Afterward, the course of the pregnancy and the condition of the delivered infant will be evaluated to determine the best treatment of the patient for her next pregnancy (if desired).

Given all of these developments, federal and state governments may decide to impose more regulations on infertility treatment in general. ART will need much stricter regulation than it has now. It is high time for the government to come up with a system governing the prescription and treatment of ART that isn't generated by the providers, who have a financial interest in it.

Many expert observers of the medical scene agree with me that government intervention of this type is long overdue. Rebecca Skloot, life sciences editor of *Popular Science* magazine, wrote on this subject recently in *The New York Times*. Her words are worth quoting at length because they offer a good summary of the situation and they represent the opinions of many reproductive health professionals who have long felt frustrated by the absence of any federal standards, support, or recourse:

> It's stunning how much attention is being paid to human cloning, given that most scientists acknowledge it may never be feasible or desirable, let alone commonplace. It's even more amazing when you consider that thousands of children are already being produced each year through potentially dangerous techniques — with scant notice from policymakers....
>
> Just within the last year [2002], a stream of studies has found that infertility treatments may carry potentially fatal risks. In March 2002, a study in the New England Journal of Medicine reported that the occurrence of major birth defects more than doubles, from 4 percent to about 9 percent, with common infertility treatments like in vitro fertilization and intercytoplasmic sperm injection — the procedure for injecting sperm directly into an egg.

So far in 2003, three more studies produced similar data: one found an increased risk of Beckwith-Wiedemann syndrome, which causes enlarged organs and childhood cancer; another found a five- to seven-fold increased risk of retinoblastoma, a malignant eye tumor....

Where is Washington in all this? Since the advent of reproductive medicine more than 30 years ago, the federal government has had almost no role in overseeing the technology or guaranteeing its safety. Despite recent studies, no governmental agency has mandated—or even argued for—further investigation into the risks of assisted reproduction. In addition, most infertility researchers and doctors aren't bound by federal regulations governing research on human subjects. As a result, no one ensures that they inform infertile patients about these safety concerns. Simply put, reproductive technologies have fallen through the regulatory cracks for decades.

The nature of the work has had much to do with this. Because developing safe infertility treatments involves human embryos at some stage—either in devising and testing technologies or in their clinical application—the field is mired in the debate over abortion. As a result, infertility doctors and researchers rarely get federal financing....The field is largely kept afloat by the billions of dollars patients spend to conceive....

If the far-off prospect of cloning can arouse such heated debate, surely the safety of current infertility methods can do the same. It took scientists decades to figure out that diethylstilbestrol, or DES, a widely used fertility drug of the 50s and 60s, caused cancer and infertility in children exposed to it in their mothers' wombs. Let's not make that mistake again. [75]

The time will come when infertility therapy will be rationed and contraindicated in certain situations because of all the potential risks and expenses involved. I believe that every aspect of infertility treatment that remains controversial should be banned from practical application until the controversy is resolved. It should have to stand the trial of double blind studies and long term follow-ups before it is passed along to patients, just like drugs and procedures in other branches of medicine.

Can we then win the battle against infertility? Certainly we can. It won't happen in one generation, but it will happen eventually. Nature's restorative powers are miraculous. But we have to cooperate with nature. Considering the superior resilience of our immune system during the second and third decades of our life, it is better for us to start having children earlier on average than we do now and preferably with better preserved reproductive tracts than we have now. Both sexes will need to rearrange their social and reproductive priorities in order for these kinds of changes to occur. Society in general will need to become more conservative about sexual mores. Only time will tell if these major shifts are possible.

I feel this is a proper place to insert my own views relating to the abortion issue, because they raise an issue that certain prospective parents may have to consider more carefully in the future. Speaking strictly as a scientist concerned about human health and the survival of the species, I would like to see fewer abortions performed on young women who get pregnant when they first become sexually active. This is, unfortunately, one of the biggest categories of women who seek and get abortions [76]. The reason I feel this way is that a woman's first child, at the onset of her sexual activity, will experience the cleanest possible uterine environment and is thus likely to be her healthiest possible child. As a result of acquired bacteria through subsequent sexual activity, future pregnancies are apt to occur in a more contaminated environment. In my opinion, this is one of the main hidden circumstances supporting the ancient "right of the first-born"—namely, that the first-born child is, generally speaking, the healthiest one. Having said this, I don't propose any legislation regarding abortion one way or the other.

I do see the possibility of controversies in the future involving a person's individual rights, as science discovers more about the full range of health and reproductive difficulties caused by horizontally and vertically transmitted bacteria. For example, one sexual partner might feel justified in suing the other for passing along an infection. And a person's medical records, pointing more clearly than they do now to possible infection-related health problems, may cause added trouble when he or she applies for insurance or employment. We already see this dilemma brewing in regard to people who are infected with HIV. We may even see people targeted for discrimination because they belong to a population group that has a higher-than-normal risk of pathogenic contamination.

* * * * *

Once again, we can only hope that human beings and human societies evolve to manage such complex developments in the best manner possible. While there may be much to cause concern in the near future, there is also bound to be much that offers new promise.

More and more over the past century, we've seen that these two trends come in a single package.

Similarly, the individual can't safely separate his or her own self-interest from the well-being of society as a whole. If we want our children and our children's children to live in a healthy world, the time to start working on it is right now.

CHAPTER 6 REFERENCES

1. Collins J. "An international survey of health economics of IVF and ICSI." *Human Reproduction Update,* 2002; 8: 365-77.
2. Roest J., Mous H.V., Zeilmaker G.H., Verhoff A. "The incidence of major clinical complications in a Dutch transport IVF program." *Human Reproduction Update,* 1996; 2: 345-53.
3. Tallo C.P., Vohr B., Oh W., Rubin L.P., Seifer D.B., Haning R.Vjr. "Maternal and neonatal morbidity associated with in vitro fertilization." *J Pediatr,* 1995; 127: 794-800.
4. Gleicher, N. "Modern obstetrical and infertility care may increase the prevalence of disease: an evolutionary concept." *Fertil Steril,* 2003; 79 (2): 249.
5. Zhang R.R., Zhao X. "The state of marriage and fertility of women born in the region of Guangxu of the Qing: a retrospective survey of the states of marriage and fertility of 90-94 year old women in Hebei province." *Chinese Journal of Population Science,* 1991; 3: 1-10.
6. Che Y., Leland J. "Infertility in Shanghai: prevalence, treatment seeking and impact." *J Obstetr Gynecol,* 2002; 22: 643-8
7. Zhang S.C., Wang H.Y., Wang J.D. "Analysis of changes in sperm quality of Chinese fertile men during 1981-1998." *Shengzui Yu Biyun,* 1999; 10: 33-9.
8. Abbotts J., Williams R., Smith G.D. "Mortality in men of Irish heritage in West Scotland." *Public Health,* 1998; 112: 229-32.
9. Swerdlow A. "Mortality and cancer incidence in Vietnamese refugees in England and Wales: a follow-up study." *International Journal of Epidemiology,* 1991; 20: 13-9.
10. Rissel C., Russel C. "Heart disease risk factors in the Vietnamese community of southwestern Sidney." *Australian Journal of Public Health,* 1993; 17: 71-3.
11. Hemminski K., Li X. "Cancer risk in Nordic immigrants and their offspring in Sweden." *European Journal of Cancer,* 2002; 38: 2428-34.
12. Gupta S. "Can environmental factors explaining the epidemiology of schizophrenia in immigrant groups." *Social Psychiatry and Psychiatric Epidemiology,* 1993; 28: 263-6.
13. Bongard S. Pogge S.F., Arslander H., Rohrmann S., Hoddapp V. "Acculturation and cardiovascular reactivity of second-generation Turkish migrants in Germany." *Journal of Psychosomatic Research,* 2002; 53: 795-803.
14. Aszalos Z., Barsi P., Vitrai J., Nagy Z. "Hypertension and cluster of risk factors in different stroke subtypes (an analysis of Hungarian patients via Budapest Stroke Data Bank)." *Journal of Human Hypertension,* 2002; 16: 495-500.

15. Jozan P. "New trend in mortality and life expectancy: epidemiologic transition in Hungary." *Orvosi Hetilap*, 2003; 144: 451-60.
16. Szabolcs O. "Cancer epidemiology in Hungary and the Bela Johan national program for the decade of health." 2003; 4: 443-52.
17. Drzewieniecka K. Dzienio K. "Mortality by sex, age and cause of death in European and highly developed extra-European countries in the years 1960-1984." *Polish Population Review*, 1993; 3: 163-88.
18. Leasure J.W. "The historical decline of fertility in Eastern Europe." *European Journal of Population*, 1992; 8: 47-75.
19. Laumann E.O., Youm Y. "Racial/ethnic group differences in the prevalence of sexually transmitted diseases in the United States: a network explanation." *Sexually Transmitted Diseases*, 1999; 26: 262-4.
20. Ness R.B., Hillier S., Richter H.E., et al. "Can known risk factors explain racial differences in the occurrence of bacterial vaginosis?" *J Natl Med Assoc* 2003; 95: 201-12.
21. CDC Report. "Healthy people 2010: Focus Area 12. Heart disease and stroke."
22. Howard G, Howard VJ. "Ethnic disparities in stroke: the scope of the problem." *Ethnicity & Disease* 2001; 11: 761-8.
23. Cooper R., Cutler J., Desvigne-Nickens P., et al. "Trends and disparities in coronary heart disease and stroke and other cardiovascular diseases in the United States: findings of the national conference on cardiovascular disease prevention." *Circulation* 2000; 19: 3137-47.
24. CDC Report. "Healthy people 2010: Focus Area 5. Diabetes."
25. McNabb W., Quinn M., Tobian J. "Diabetes in African American women: the silent epidemic." *Women's Health*, 1997; 3: 275-300.
26. Raddy S., Shapiro M., Morton R. Jr., Brawley OW. "Prostate cancer in blacks and white Americans." *Cancer and Metastasis Reviews*, 2003; 22: 83-6.
27. Ademuyiwa F.O., Olepado O.I. "Racial differences in genetic factors associated with breast cancer." *Cancer Metastasis Rev*, 2003; 22: 47-53.
28. Gadgeel S.M., Kalemkerian G.P. "Racial differences in lung cancer." *Cancer Metastasis Rev* 2003; 22: 39-46.
29. MacDorman M.F., Minino A.M., Strobino D.M., Guyer B. "Annual summary of vital statistics—2001." *Pediatrics*, 2002; 110: 1037-52.
30. Blackmore-Prince C, et al. "Racial differences in the patterns of singleton preterm deliveries in the 1998 National Maternal and Infant Health Survey." *Maternal and Child Health Journal*, 1999; 3: 189-97.
31. MacKay A.P., Berg C.J., Atrash .H.K. "Pregnancy-related mortality from preeclampsia and eclampsia." *Obstet Gynecol*, 2001; 97: 533-8.
32. Emmanuel I., Leisenring W., Williams M.A., Kimpo C., et al. "The Washington State Intergenerational Study of Birth Outcomes: methodology and some comparisons of maternal birth weight and gestation in four ethnic groups." *Pediatric and Perinatal Epidemiology*, 2000; 13: 378-80.

33. Fiscella K. "Race, perinatal outcome and amniotic infection." *Obstetrical & Gynecological Survey,* 1996; 51: 60-6.

34. Collins J.W. Jr. "Disparate black and white neonatal mortality rates among infants of normal birth weight in Chicago: a population study." *J Pediatr,* 1992; 120: 954-60.

35. Adams C.D., Kelly M.L., McCarthy M. "The Adolescent Behavior Checklist: development and initial psychometric properties of a self-report measure for adolescent with ADHD." *Journal of Clinical Child Psychology,* 1997; 26: 77-86.

36. Avila W.S., Rossi E.G., Ramires J.A., et al. "Pregnancy with heart disease: experience with 1,000 cases." *Clinical Cardiology,* 2003 26: 135-42.

37. Smulian J.C., Ananth C.V., Vintzileos A.M., Scorza W.E., Knuppel R.A. "Fetal death in the United States. Influence of high-risk conditions and implications for management." *Obstet Gynecol,* 2002; 100: 1183-9.

38. Saran M. "The ethics of cloning and human embryo research." *Princeton Journal of Bioethics* 2002; 5: 25-36.

39. Schillberg S., Fischer R., Emans N. "Molecular farming of recombinant antibodies in plants." *Cellular and Molecular Life Sciences,* 2003; 60: 433-45.

40. Mitalipov S.M., Wolf D.P. "Mammalian cloning: possibilities and threats." *Annals of Medicine,* 2000; 32: 462-8.

41. Rubanyi G.M. "The future of human gene therapy." *Molecular Aspects of Medicine* 2001; 22: 113-42.

42. ADA. "Economic consequences of diabetes mellitus in the US in 1997." *Diabetes Care* 1998; 21: 296-306.

43. Leonard P., Sur S. "Asthma: future directions." *Med Clin North Am,* 2002; 86: 1131-56.

44. Shell E.R. *Interior Design,* 2002 (Dec), pp. 49-52.

45. Lumey L.H. "Decreased birth weight in infants after maternal in utero exposure to the Dutch famine of 1944-1945." *Pediat Perinat Epid,* 1992; 6: 240-253.

46. Smith C.A. "The effect of wartime starvation in Holland upon pregnancy and its product." *Am J Obstet Gynecol,* 1947; 53: 599-608.

47. Rich-Edwards, J.W., et al. "Birth weight and risk of cardiovascular disease of women followed up since 1976." *British Medical Journal,* 1997; 315: 396-400.

48. Stein C.E., et al. "Fetal growth and coronary heart disease in South India." *Lancet* 1996; 348: 1269-1273.

49. Martyn C.N., et al. "Mothers' pelvic size, fetal growth and death from stroke and coronary heart disease in the UK." *Lancet,* 1996; 348: 1264-1268.

50. Curham, GC et al. "Birth weight and adult hypertension and diabetes mellitus in US men." *American Journal of Hypertension* 1996; 9: 11 (Abstract).

51. Halws C.N. "Fetal and infant growth and impaired glucose tolerance in adulthood: The Thrifty Phenotype hypothesis revisited." *Acta Paediatrica Supplementum,* 1997; 422: 73-77.
52. Lithell H.O., et al. "Relation of size at birth to non-insulin dependent diabetes and insulin concentrations in men aged 50-60." *Br Med J,* 1996; 312: 406-410.
53. Ravelli G.P. "Obesity in young men after famine exposure in utero and early infancy." *N Eng J Med,* 1976; 295: 34.
54. Stanner S.A., et al. "Does malnutrition in utero determines diabetes and coronary heart disease in adulthood? Results from the Leningrad siege study, a cross sectional study." *Brit Med J* 1997; 315: 1342-1349.
55. Ravelli A.C.J., et al. "Glucose tolerance in adults after prenatal exposure to famine." *Lancet* 1998; 351: 173-177.
56. Lumey L.H., Stein A.D. "In utero exposure to famine and subsequent fertility: The Dutch Famine Birth Cohort Study." *Am J Public Health,* 1997; 87: 1962-6.
57. Laitman C.J. "DES exposure and the aging mothers and daughters." *Current Women's Health Reports,* 2002; 2: 390-3.
58. Mei Z., Grimmer-Strawn L.M., Scanlon K.S. "Does overweight in infancy persist though the preschool years? An analysis of CDC Pediatric Nutrition Surveillance data." *Soc Prevent Med,* 2003; 48(3): 161-7.
59. Reaven G.M. "Importance of identifying the overweight patient who will benefit the most by losing weight." *Annals of Internal Medicine,* 2003; 138: 420-3.
60. Jensen D.M., Damm P., Sorensen B., Molsted-Pedersen L., Westergaard J.G., Ovesen P., Beck-Nielsen H. "Pregnancy outcome and pregnancy body mass index in 2459 glucose-tolerant Danish women." *Am J Obstet Gynecol,* 2003; 189(1): 239-44.
61. O'Brien T.E., Ray J.G., Chan W.S. "Maternal body mass index and the risk of preeclampsia: a systemic overview." *Epidemiology* 2003; 14(3): 368-74.
62. Watkins M.L., Rasmussen S.A., Honein M.A., Botto L.D.,. Moore C.A. "Maternal obesity and risk for birth defects." *Pediatrics* 2003; 111(5/2): 1152-8.
63. Van der spuy Z.M., Jacobs H.S. "Weight reduction, fertility and contraception." *IPPF Medical Bulletin,* 1983; 17: 2-4
64. Chapieski M.L., Evankovich K.D. "Bahavioral effects of prematurity." *Seminars in Perinatology* 1997; 21(3): 221-39.
65. Caroll C.S., et al. "Vaginal birth after cesarean section versus elective repeat cesarean delivery: Weight –based outcome." *Am J Obstet Gynecol* 2003; 188: 1516-20. (High infectious mortality and less success in VBAC)
66. Jensen D.M., et al. "Pregnancy outcome and pregnancy body mass index in 2459 glucose-tolerant Danish women." *Am J Obstetr Gynecol* 2003; 189: 239-44. (HBP, C/S induction, macrosomia)

67. Rashid M.N., Fuentes F., Touchon R.C., Wehner P.S. "Obesity and the risk for cardiovascular disease." *Preventive Cardiology,* 2003; 6: 42-7. (clear association)
68. Hall J.E. "The kidney, hypertension and obesity." *Hypertension* 2003; 41: 625-33. (Hypertension associated with obesity)
69. Qiu C., Williams M.A., Leisenring W.M., et al. "Family history of hypertension and type 2 diabetes in relation to preeclampsia risk." *Hypertension* 2003; 41: 408-13. (Father mother or sibling HBP Diabetes increases the risk for preeclampsia)
70. Gillman M.W., Rifas-Shiman S., Berkey C.S., et al. "Maternal gestational diabetes, birth weight and adolescent obesity." *Pediatrics* 2003; 111: 221-6. (GDM babies are more likely overweight in adolescence)
71. Marchesini G., et al. "Nonalcoholic fatty liver, steatohepatitis and the metabolic syndrome." *Hepatology* 2003; 37: 917-23.
72. Norman R.J., Clark A.M. "Obesity and reproductive disorder: a review." *Reproduction, Fertility, and Development* 1998; 10: 55-63.
73. Castello E.J., Mustillo S., Erkanli A., Keeler G., Angold A. "Prevalence and development of psychiatric disorders in childhood and adolescence." *Archives of General Psychiatry* 2003; 60: 837-33.
74. Robinson I.M., Skaer T.L., Sclar D.A., Galin R.S. "Is attention deficit hyperactivity disorder increasing among girls in the US? Trends in diagnosis and the prescribing of stimulants." *CNS Drugs* 2002; 16: 129-37.
75. Skloot, Rebecca L. "The Other Baby Experiment," *The New York Times,* February 22, 2003, p. A17.
76. CDC Surveillance Summaries. "Abortion Surveillance—United States, 1999." 2002; 51(SS09): 1-28.

CHAPTER 7

SELF-ASSESSMENT: YOUR OWN FERTILITY AND HEALTH RISKS

The secret to mastering all the big challenges we encounter rests in our courage to look within. The more we endeavor to learn who we truly are, beginning on the most physical level, the more we know about life in general and the wiser we are in living it.

—Dr. Jonas Salk

Most likely, you grew up expecting that the path to parenthood would be an easy one. During your early adolescence, your parents might have warned you that it was too easy for your own good, and you needed to take special care not to create an unwanted pregnancy. As an adult, you may have previously conceived and given birth to a child with no trouble, thus confirming your belief that the process should be smooth and simple.

Now, facing infertility, you may understandably have trouble accepting that the path to parenthood might be full of twists and much longer than you ever thought it would be. From a psychological point of view, this situation can be one of the most agonizing that a human being can face. It seems unfair, illogical, a betrayal of the body and inspires all sorts of unwanted feelings of guilt, shame, fear, and frustration. No wonder many infertile couples lean from the start toward choosing ART-based approaches to the problem and, directly or indirectly, send signals of this inclination to their doctor. If nothing else, they appear to offer the quickest route to the desired end. And even if they don't, even if they fail time and again, actually making the process longer than more conservative treatment might have taken, they allow everyone involved to skip over the more demanding, emotionally-charged business of pinning down what is wrong internally and then doing whatever is necessary to make it right again.

After reading this book I hope you will choose to take on this demanding but ultimately rewarding business first, despite any pressures you and your physician may feel to move immediately toward ART solutions. For the sake of yourself, your family, and your future child, it makes sense to take the time and make the effort to identify and treat the cause of your infertility before you go any further. This means overcoming any natural reluctance you have not only to proceed more slowly toward conception, but also to probe more deeply into your past reproductive history, to talk with family members about your infertility, to question doctors about their decisions, or to assume a more active role in managing your health care.

Why is this book urging you to take the road less traveled? Because it brings the greatest rewards. It is the surest path toward regaining your own health and having a healthy child, whether or not you eventually rely on ART. It also gives you a great deal of otherwise unattainable information about what to expect in the future regarding your overall health and that of your baby.

What can I do to assist you along the way? In this chapter you will find self-assessment tools that will help you examine your past more thoroughly for possible causes of infertility and communication guidelines that will help you talk more effectively with key family members and doctors, so that they can respond more wholeheartedly to your needs.

PREPARING TO CONSULT A DOCTOR

Typically people go to a doctor and complain about a physical problem they are having, and then they leave it up to the doctor to do all the investigative and decision-making work. Our culture reinforces this pattern. "Back off and let an expert handle it!" is our credo for everything from car trouble and financial planning to marital discord and grief counseling.

In the case of a physical illness or incapacity, it certainly does make sense to solicit the help of qualified professionals, given the highly complex nature of modern medicine, but leaving them "free" to do everything is foolish and even dangerous. It's as if you were handicapping them from the start. Yes, turning it all over to them relieves you of having to deal with the problem in anything but a passive way ("passive" having the same linguistic origin as "patient"). Unfortunately, however, it also means depriving them—and yourself—of your own irreplaceable expertise in the matter.

In the case of infertility in particular, you know more than anyone else about how it has manifested itself in your body, your mind, and your lifestyle. You also know more than anyone else about your history, your situation now, and your desires for the future. To ensure that you get the most effective and efficient treatment available, you need to take control of the treatment process, offering as much constructive input as you can along the way and equipping yourself to be the best "final decision-maker" possible regarding which treatment options to pursue.

At the end of this chapter are six questionnaires that can assist you and your partner to do most of the vitally important groundwork for good infertility treatment—the history-taking itself. Every doctor and clinic in the field requires a certain amount of history-taking as a first step. The questionnaires here, designed for your own use, paint an even more thorough background picture. They not only give you a concise overview of the major illnesses and reproductive problems you have experienced, but also offer clues about pathogenic infections you may have acquired either horizontally or vertically and, therefore, about wide-ranging health risks you may have in the future. Altogether they cover the general and reproductive health history of yourself and your partner and, branching out from there, all related siblings, parents, and grandparents (you may be unable to get full information about all these people, but any information you can get will help). More specific directions on how to complete, interpret, and utilize the questionnaires appear later in the chapter.

To answer as many questions as you can, you will probably need to do a certain amount of research on your own and talk with other knowledgeable family members. Regrettably, many people do not keep good records of the illnesses they have had and how they were treated—a wealth of data that can benefit both themselves and their relatives. If you are one of these people, it is not too late to start right now.

Everyone should keep a personal medical file just like they do a photo album or a record of car maintenance. In this age of specialization, when we tend to see one or more different doctors for each significant illness we experience, a record of this kind can serve as the only centralized source of medical information about ourselves. In it should go copies of medical records (which we should obtain for every major illness), contact information for the relevant doctors and service institutions, prescription drug labels, and even subjective remarks about anything experienced or learned during the illness and its treatment.

If you have already kept such a record for some time, it will assist you in answering the questionnaires. If you haven't, and you don't know, can't recall, or have no record of various details in your health history—particularly surrounding your birth—you can try obtaining this information from the doctors, clinics, or hospitals involved, assuming you know them and they are still in operation. Often, however, this kind of search leads nowhere: medical records in such offices are not kept forever, are frequently relocated, and can easily get lost or destroyed. In this situation, your only recourse is to seek input from family members who may have it: especially your parents and siblings, whom you will most likely need to interview anyway in order to get the requisite details of their own health histories.

Many infertile individuals or couples find it awkward or embarrassing to discuss their conception-related problems with family members or, for that matter, to start a two-way conversation with them about anything having to do with sex, reproduction, or even illness in general. Nevertheless, it is best if the whole family knows about the situation and, with your permission, can get constructively involved in it.

This kind of sharing not only ends unwanted speculation ("Why aren't they having a baby?") but also circulates health-related information that may make a vital difference to other family members who experience related difficulties in the future. In addition, it enables people who care about you to offer valuable love and support right from the start. Let me give you some tips for handling such conversations.

TALKING WITH FAMILY AND FRIENDS

- If possible, try to meet one-on-one with individuals. Keep in mind that interviewing two people separately about the same issue can be very informative about possible areas of ambiguity.

- Target whom to interview first. Consider beginning with the most knowledgeable person about family health history matters, but also take into account the person you can approach most comfortably. Talking with the latter first, whether or not this person is the best informed on the topic, may build your confidence and sharpen your interview skills before you go any further. Also think about who might know the best way to approach a more difficult interviewee. For example, speaking first with a particular brother, sister, or family friend might yield good advice on how to go about interviewing your mother.

- Prepare in advance by reviewing all the questionnaires and asking yourself:

  ° "What do I already know—or think I know—regarding this person's health/reproductive history [assuming your interviewee is a sibling, parent, or grandparent]?" You want to check with this person to make sure your current understanding is accurate and complete.

  ° "What might this person know about the health/reproductive history of any of the other individuals involved [yourself, your siblings, your parents, your grandparents]?" You especially want to fill in places in the questionnaires where you currently have no information.

  ° "What suggestions might this person have for contacting other primary interviewees and knowledgeable individuals or for getting relevant information from other sources?"

- Schedule your talk with each person in advance. After doing the appropriate preparation (see above), tell him or her that you'd like to talk about some important matters relating to the family's health history. Mutually choose a time, place, and situation comfortable for both of you and free from disturbance or distraction. If you think the other person would enjoy reading this book beforehand, encourage it. Otherwise, it isn't necessary.

- When opening the interview (or describing it ahead of time, if appropriate), be brief and to the point. You don't need to go into details about, for example, horizontal or vertical transmission or even about your own case of infertility unless the interviewee expresses interest or you feel compelled to discuss these matters in the spirit of reciprocity. Otherwise, details of this nature can be intimidating, making the interviewee think he or she has to respond more authoritatively or scientifically than necessary. An early mention of vertical transmission can even make some parents become defensive. A good all-purpose opener is something like, "I'm seeking therapy for possible infertility. The first step is to get as much information as I can about the general health and reproductive history of close blood relatives. Any illness or reproductive difficulty that I've had, or that has occurred in the last two generations in my family, could have a bearing on my ability to have a child."

- When talking with the other person, stay focused on the subject matter of the questionnaires. Don't divide your attention by simultaneously, for example, eating a meal, playing cards, or taking a walk. Take written notes even if you also use a tape recorder, just in case the tape fails.

- Be sure to allow your interviewee plenty of time to answer a question after you have posed it. Avoid interrupting or bringing a silence to a premature close. Go beyond "yes" or "no" answers to establish, for example, the severity or duration of a particular illness or condition, the explanation for it, and the reaction to it on an emotional or practical level. Encourage your interviewee to get back to you with any information he or she can't recall or locate on the spot.

- Besides completing the questionnaires, another vitally important preparatory step is to read as much literature as you can about infertility and its causes and treatments. This background will help you to better understand your own case and make your discussion with doctors more productive. An excellent source for the latest information is the Internet, but be careful to pick sites that have good credentials or that are suggested to you by reliable people. Here are sites I can recommend to get you started:

- www.infertilitytimes.com (Infertility Times Database)

- www.inciid.org (International Council on Infertility Information Dissemination)

- www.resolve.org (National Infertility Association)

- www.americaninfertility.org (American Infertility Association)

- www.nlm.nih.org/medlineplus/infertility.html (National Institute of Children's Health and Human Development)

- www.fertilitysolution.com Official website of The MacLeod Laboratory.

- www.IVFconnections.com Open forum for patients undergoing IVF treatment.

- www.Fertilethoughts.com One of the largest open forums for all infertile patients.

CHOOSING OR CHANGING A DOCTOR

For the treatment of a complicated condition like infertility, which involves professional expertise in reproductive medicine, endocrinology, and microbiology, a couple is better off going to a reputable medical center or clinic. To qualify individual doctors, check the following issues through direct communication with the doctor, research with the center or clinic's administrative staff, or your own investigation of literature and websites:

- What is the doctor's educational background and training?

- How long has the doctor practiced in his or her current capacity?

- With what hospital, organizations, and institutions is the doctor professionally affiliated?

- What kind of services can this doctor and his/her clinic or center provide?

- What are the doctor's special areas of expertise?

- How extensive is the doctor's experience with the kind of infertility problem(s) you're experiencing and with patients of your age and background?

- What (if anything) has the doctor written on the subject?

In addition, you may find it helpful to discuss clinic, center, and doctor recommendations with others you know and trust who have undergone or are undergoing treatment for infertility.

During your initial interview with a doctor and throughout the course of your therapy, you might consider changing doctors if you can't answer "yes" to any of the following questions:

- Is the doctor good at explaining things?

- Given that you may have difficulty talking with doctors in general, is it relatively easy to talk with this doctor?

- Given that the doctor may not be able to give definite answers to some questions, does he or she answer your questions clearly, thoughtfully, and in a timely fashion?

- Does the doctor take into proper account your concerns, preferences, opinions, and emotional feelings?

- Does the doctor give you his or her full attention and allow sufficient time for individual consultations?

- Given the fact that your case may be difficult or your own emotional response to it may be complicated, does the doctor help you to feel relatively confident about what is happening?

CONSULTING A DOCTOR

As I mentioned earlier, doctors can be intimidating to patients simply because our culture has conditioned us to put ourselves entirely in their hands and not to question what they do. In fact, just because a person has a medical degree doesn't mean he or she knows more than you do about your infertility or even the latest thinking on various aspects of infertility, assuming you have done the background research suggested above. Some doctors don't have time to keep up with the literature in all areas of their field. Also, you know more about your own health history and your own experience of infertility-related problems to date than someone you are consulting for the first time.

The questionnaire answers and the background information you have researched are for your own benefit. It's not a good idea merely to hand your doctor a file of all this material to read. Instead, use it to determine what you will eventually ask the doctor to do for you. Having accumulated and considered this material on your own, review it again before talking with the doctor, and isolate the following details:

- Drawing on what you have learned from the questionnaires, what events in your own reproductive history concern you the most as possible indicators that you might be infected with pathogens? You don't need to involve your doctor in a discussion of complex issues relating to vertical transmission or the possible connection between other major health problems and infertility. It is more important to zero in on certain episodes in your past that are important to discuss and will lead to a better understanding of the primary causes of your infertility.

- Drawing on what you have learned from reviewing infertility literature, what parallels do you see between your own experience and the experiences they describe? For discussion purposes with your doctor, choose what you consider to be the strongest parallels in terms of case histories or symptom descriptions.

When you consult a doctor, you want to present your case concisely. You want to build a logical foundation, drawing on your own reproductive health experience, to serve as the basis for asking particular questions. Here is a brief example of how such a case-presentation may start:

"I suffer from secondary infertility. My first conception was easy but now four years have gone by and I cannot get pregnant again." From here you should focus on any abnormal or unusual occurrences during the pregnancy and delivery and how close the delivery was to the actual due date. From there you will move on to detail adverse medical conditions in your child and recall all changes that took place in your own pelvis following delivery. Having read this book you will probably list a number of changes that have developed and these will more than likely direct you straight to an infectious cause behind the secondary infertility. If you did your exploratory work diligently and analyzed your families' medical and reproductive histories you can even pinpoint when the pathogens entered the family line. When you have finished, the doctor will take over and draw up a plan of action.

During the course of your interactions with the doctor, be willing to take the initiative whenever you feel it is necessary. If your doctor orders a course of action or a set of tests, don't be afraid to ask questions about whatever is being done or not done, for example: "Why is this test being ordered?" "How will it be accomplished?" "What does it cost?" "When and how will I know the results?" "Why are we ignoring my husband's history of prostatitis?" "How was my tubal damage caused?"

Above all, never be afraid to advocate in favor of antibiotic therapy, the most natural mode of treating infertility. If you suspect it is being overlooked, ask, "Why are we bypassing antibiotic therapy?" If, for example, you have undergone any kind of adverse hormonal change following your pregnancy, a two- or three-week course of a culture specific, broad-spectrum antibiotic such as Doxycyline, Augmentin, or Erythromycin could reverse the change.

The most effective way to make your request for antibiotic therapy is to first bring up your own experience relating to the request (that is, the reproductive problem or history involved), then to probe for what the doctor is thinking, and finally, after acknowledging the doctor's input, to tell him or her the course you want to pursue. If you need more time to reach a final decision, by all means take it, assuming you don't postpone treatment for too long a period.

In another scenario, before you had the chance to read my book for example, suppose that your doctor, who favors hormone stimulation as a therapy, has given you Pergonal shots followed by three intrauterine inseminations (IUI), and the cycle failed. Afterward, during a post-failure conference, you might say, "You know, I felt funny after the inseminations. My abdomen felt bloated, my breasts felt sore, and I was very irritable. I also noticed some staining midway through the cycle."

Your doctor might say, "Those are classic symptoms of luteal phase defect [sluggish hormone support of the second half of the cycle]. Next time, I'll give you more Pergonal and some Progesterone support."

Although your doctor may be right in diagnosing the situation as luteal phase defect, and although the kind of hormone therapy he suggests is a standard way of addressing the problem, you suspect that the source of the problem is most likely pathogenic. Furthermore, you want to get to the source of the problem in the most natural way possible. Therefore, you should say something like, "I realize that luteal phase defect is probably what's happening. But I don't want to go through another round of hormonal stimulation right now. I think I've got an infection. Why don't we do some testing for bacteria?"

Your doctor might override this request by responding, "Well, we could test your cervical mucus, but I don't think that's necessary. After all, the inseminations are made above the cervix."

Unfortunately, many highly qualified, compassionate, and well-meaning doctors who are oriented toward technological solutions would choose inseminations for their patients, and, therefore, tend to dismiss antibiotic therapy prematurely. In fact, I regret having to say that it's almost a conflict of interest these days for doctors and clinics not to resort to the most sophisticated technological approaches whenever they are feasible. Clinics are set up to utilize them, and, to be honest, the clinics need the money that comes from them to pay for their investment in the technology.

As a result, when you are faced with this kind of contradictory response from a doctor, you have an obligation to yourself to speak up for what you think is right. You need to say something like, "No, it's my reproductive tract, and I want to make sure it is clean. I won't go another step until we address any possible infection."

Let's assume you are a woman in your mid-thirties, who is about ready to start a family. As you reconstruct your early post-menarche years, it occurs to you that you were menstruating normally until age 18, but from then on your periods became irregular and you were troubled with recurrent ovarian cysts. Not much later severe PMS symptoms started and by the time you were twenty years old you had signs of full-blown endometriosis. After consulting several specialists, you were placed on long-term birth control pills. Subsequently, your menstruation became regular, your PMS symptoms abated, and the violent cramps preceding your periods became tolerable.

Now that you have read the book and realize that all these events happened before you ever engaged in sexual activity, you can exclude the possibility that your problems were due to a horizontally-transmitted infection. Instead, you know that the infection was acquired vertically. The information you have gathered on your own can even give you a rough idea of how difficult it may be to fix the problem. However, your first job is to convince your doctor that you believe an infection may be the source of your problems, not to go into a long explanation of horizontal and vertical transmission.

Start by expressing your concern that an acidic vagina or recurring yeast infections may be making the area too hostile to sperms. Ask for an evaluation and insist that it include bacteria cultures. If your request for cultures is declined or brushed aside, ask the doctor to check for bacterial vaginosis. The chances are very high you will have it. If the diagnosis of bacterial vaginosis is not made at that time, insist on performing a post-coital test (PC).

During the month while you are having the PC test, request a day three hormone evaluation for FSH, LH, and estradiol. My guess is that your hormone values will be in the "acceptable" range—nothing too good and nothing too bad—so the situation is workable. The PC test in general tends to be neglected by the profession and practiced correctly by only a few physicians. You should be in charge of timing your ovulation, so that you know the optimum time for getting a specimen. You should also insist on looking into the microscope yourself to see if a large number of sperm are swimming linearly (a sign that the mucus is clean and healthy). Given the history I've described above, I predict it will be hard to find living, moving cells in the specimen, and white blood cells will be obliterating the view. Your insistence has paid off—the infectious problem has been located!

Measuring the uterine lining and documenting the ovulatory follicle are also integral parts of a well-conducted PC, so you should be sure that your doctor does these things. When your doctor reports the results, make a note of how thick the lining is in millimeters and whether it has developed a properly layered structure. This information will give you a baseline for evaluating subsequent cycles. Photographs of the lining can assist you immensely in the future.

For the time being you should decline artificial insemination, which, regrettably, is suggested routinely at this point by many doctors. Instead, insists on a course of antibiotics, since the white blood cells in your specimen are bothersome. You can be confident that the next month, following the completion of antibiotic therapy, all measured parameters, including the hormone studies, will show improvements.

Thanks to the positive way your train of analysis is working, this is the time you can expect a doctor to begin showing genuine interest in it. If your personal assessment of your family history, using the questionnaires in this book, indicates the presence of serious, stubborn bacteria in your family history, you are likely to experience a reversal of the improvements in your reproductive health within one month. If that happens, I encourage you to ask for a stronger course of antibiotic therapy: one that lasts longer and features either a combination of oral antibiotics or intravenous antibiotic therapy.

If your first antibiotic course yields to a pregnancy, you need to make sure that that pregnancy isn't compromised by a resurging infection. Whether or not post-conceptional cultures are done, you and your doctor should analyze carefully whether an infection still persists and, if you feel there is this possibility, you should consider having post-conceptional antibiotic therapy. Based on the progress you have already made by following your own recommendations, you will probably not meet much resistance from the doctor when you ask for a two-week course of safe, oral antibiotics.

There are a number of events that can lead to subsequent reproductive problems requiring antibiotic therapy. Among them are the following:

- prior to menarche (the onset of menstruation): any profuse vaginal discharge or recurring bladder infections (signs that an infection has been vertically transferred)

- post menarche, before sexual activity:

  ○ a normally occurring period that becomes irregular, or amenorrhea developing within a few years

- ° the development of ovarian cysts
- ° the development of endometriosis
- post menarche, after sexual activity begins:
  - ° all of the above
  - ° extended use of IUD
  - ° drastically changed menstrual flow after discontinuation of birth control pills
  - ° rapidly changing menstrual flow following discontinuation of barrier type birth control method
  - ° rapidly worsening PMS symptoms with unprotected intercourse
  - ° developing infections in any part of the reproductive canal during protected or unprotected intercourse.
- during fertility work:
  - ° any of the above developing during ART procedures
  - ° rapidly rising day-three FSH
  - ° thin, resistant endometrium
  - ° rapidly developing ovarian resistance to gonadotropins
  - ° repeatedly failed IVF cycles
- pregnancy and delivery events:
  - ° all forms of miscarriages and ectopic pregnancies
  - ° incompetent cervix
  - ° preeclampsia
  - ° any form of premature labor or delivery
  - ° the delivery of a sickly child

Here are some other suggestions for consulting with doctors:

- As much as possible, both you and your partner should be involved in every consultation with a doctor, including both office visits and telephone calls. This strategy helps ensure that both of you have a full and accurate understanding of the case and can work together to get the kind of treatment you prefer. It also better enables the two of you to support each other emotionally both during and between consultations.

• Prepare for each meeting by listing your questions. Use this list as a personal reminder of what to say, not as a document to give to the doctor in place of asking him or her directly. Conversation is a much more effective communication tool in this kind of situation.

• Make written notes even if you use a tape recorder during consultations. Keep the notes in a file.

• Ask for copies of medical records as they become available. Keep these records in the same file as the notes.

FILLING IN THE QUESTIONNAIRES

Please read through and, as much as possible, complete the six questionnaires below. Ask your partner to do the same. To facilitate the process or to preserve a clean copy of each questionnaire, you may want to photocopy the questionnaires in the book and then mark your photocopies. Otherwise, simply mark the questionnaires in the book and use extra sheets to record any notes relating to specific questions.

Your response to the questionnaires will provide you and (by way of your spoken report) any doctors you consult with background information about possible sources or signs of infertility in your past. In addition, you can score your responses to these questionnaires and get a working estimate of your overall infertility risk as a couple: LOW, MEDIUM, or HIGH. In addition, you and your partner individually can review the history of major illnesses in your respective families, especially the illnesses linked in this book with vertical transmission, to get a sense of what other health risks you may be facing in future years.

Here are brief descriptions of what the six questionnaires cover:

Personal Background Information: You and Your Partner: events in both your physical, medical, and sexual histories that may have a bearing on your current infertility.

General Health History: You and Your Partner: major illnesses experienced by you and your partner.

Reproductive Health and Fertility History: You, Your Partner, and Parents: incidents of fertility, infertility, or pregnancy-birth-post-partum complications experienced by: [1] your parents and your partner's parents, and [2] the siblings of your parents and your partner's parents; also illnesses you and your partner had at birth or during infancy.

Reproductive Health and Fertility History: Siblings: incidents of fertility, infertility, or pregnancy-birth-postpartum complications experienced by your siblings and your partner's siblings and their partners.

General Health History: Parents: major illnesses experienced by your parents and your partner's parents.

General Health History: Grandparents: major illnesses experienced by your grandparents and your partner's grandparents.

Directions for completing all the questionnaires appear at the bottom of the introductory page. When you finish filling in all the questionnaires to the best of your ability, add the scores you and your partner received for questionnaires #1 through #6. The combined figure tells you as a couple what your personal infertility risk factor is according to the following scale:

41 AND ABOVE = HIGH

20-40 = MEDIUM

0-19 = LOW

As you complete the questionnaires, please bear in mind these facts:

• The risk factor is only an estimate of your chance of being infertile. It does not by any means represent a predictor or a final judgment. Instead, it provides the valuable service of helping you (and, through your report, your doctor) better determine the need for certain diagnostic and treatment options so that you and your partner eventually have the greatest possibility of producing a healthy baby.

- You don't have to answer every question in order for the scoring to have validity. In my own experience of history-taking with patients, very few are able to respond to every question raised.

Although many different avenues of inquiry are pursued in the questionnaires, there are a limited number of causes for concern that scientists know to be especially significant. The questionnaires are constructed so that these particular causes—if they exist in one's family line—are most likely to be identified by the majority of individuals seeking help.

If you are not able to answer most of the questions and still come up with a HIGH risk factor, you will not change this factor by filling in the unknowns. However, the more you can research and find out the answers to what you don't know, the better informed you will be when you seek infertility therapy.

If you cannot answer most or even half of the questions and come up with a MEDIUM or LOW risk factor, then you will definitely want to do more research into the areas where you are uncertain. With a few more answers, you may actually learn that you have a HIGH risk factor, which is something you need to know.

- Because of the generational time spans involved, you may be unable to provide any answers for questionnaire #6, General Health History: Grandparents. Again, this doesn't invalidate your final score.

Regardless of what broad category truly characterizes your risk—HIGH, MEDIUM, or LOW, it is almost certain to show up in a review of your own and your partner's histories. If you are unable to provide answers for questionnaire #6, it will provide more confirmation, added information, and a more refined numerical score.

* * *

Keep investigating the matters raised in these questionnaires beyond your initial review and scoring. Look up old records. Interview family members and close personal friends of the family. The more you find out, the more effective your diagnosis and treatment can be.

The path you take toward giving birth to a healthy baby may not be as smooth or short as you had hoped it would be. And, realistically speaking, you have to remain prepared to accept the possibility that you won't be able to achieve your desired outcome. In any case, the path itself is worth taking as carefully and responsibly as you can. You will learn a great deal about yourself along the way, and you will be reassured knowing that you did the best you were capable of doing. I sincerely wish you good health and a good journey.

SELF EVALUATION QUESTIONNAIRES

1. Personal Background Information: You and Your Partner
Factors in your and your partner's physical, medical, sexual, and reproductive histories that may have a bearing on your currant infertility.

2. General Health Histories: You and Your Partner
Major illnesses experienced by you and your partner.

3. Reproductive Health and Fertility Histories: You, Your Partner, and Parents
Incidents of fertility, infertility, or pregnancy-birth-postpartum complications experienced by:
   a. you and your partner's parents and
   b. the siblings of you and your partner's parents.
   Illnesses you and your partner had at birth or during infancy.

4. Reproductive Health and Fertility Histories: Siblings
Incidents of fertility, infertility, or pregnancy-birth-postpartum complications experienced by you and your partner's siblings and parents.

5. General Health Histories: Parents
Major illnesses experienced by your and your partner's parents.

6. General Health Histories: Grandparents
Major illnesses experienced by your and your partner's grandparents.

DIRECTIONS:

Following each questions, there are "yes," "no," and "I don't know" choices. Mark the corresponding squares. When you have completed the questionnaire, add all the numbers next to the "yes squares" for your total score.

1. Personal Background Information: You and Your Partner

a. To be completed by wife/female partner

Am I from a small family (1 or 2 children) or am I the only child?
.... Yes 1 | No | I don't know. |
Did I enter puberty late? .... Yes 2 | No | I don't know. |
Do I have irregular periods? .... Yes 2 | No | I don't know. |
Do I have unusually painful period pains or PMS?.... Yes 2 | No | I don't know. |
Was any congenital abnormality ever mentioned? .... Yes 1 | No | I don't know. |
Any abnormal Pap smears?........................ Yes 2 | No | I don't know. |
Was I sexually active without a condom? .... Yes 1 | No | I don't know. |
Did I have genital-tract infections, treated or untreated?
.... Yes 2 | No | I don't know. |
Did any of my previous partners develop genital-tract infections while with me?
.... Yes 2 | No | I don't know. |
Was I with someone for a long time and, despite irregular use of birth control, no
   pregnancy occurred?............................ Yes 2 | No | I don't know. |
Did any pregnancy end with an abortion or delivery that was followed by
   significant changes in menstrual flow quantity, pattern, color, and/or interval
   or associated pain and PMS?...................... Yes 3 | No | I don't know. |
Did I carry a complicated pregnancy and did I give birth to a sickly child?
.... Yes 3 | No | I don't know. |
Did I develop allergies, asthma, uncontrolled weight gain and/or a thyroid
   problem following a previous delivery or abortion?.. Yes 2 | No | I don't know. |
Did I suffer from an unduly long postpartum/abortion depression?
.... Yes 1 | No | I don't know. |
Did I need psychiatric therapy after such an event? ... Yes 1 | No | I don't know. |
Did a previous relationship break up because I could not control my moods/
   feelings/responses following an abortion/delivery? .. Yes 1 | No | I don't know. |
Did I lose interest in sex after such an event?........ Yes 1 | No | I don't know. |
Did I become alienated from my partner, children, parents or friends after a
   pregnancy-related event?........................ Yes 1 | No | I don't know. |
Did I have an intervening chronic illness? .... Yes 1 | No | I don't know. |
Any hospital stays, with or without surgery? .... Yes 1 | No | I don't know. |
Any pelvic or abdominal surgery?.................. Yes 1 | No | I don't know. |
Any cervical procedures for infections, precancerous conditions?
.... Yes 1 | No | I don't know. |
Any surgery to correct congenital genito-urinary tract abnormality?
.... Yes 2 | No | I don't know. |
Did I abuse drugs, alcohol, or nicotine? .... Yes 1 | No | I don't know. |
Did I use anabolic steroids for a long period of time? . Yes 1 | No | I don't know. |
Am I bulimic?.................................... Yes 1 | No | I don't know. |
Did I lose or gain weight recently?................. Yes 1 | No | I don't know. |
Was I excessively obese before or ever after puberty?.. Yes 1 | No | I don't know. |
Am I on any drugs for the treatment of a chronic condition?
.... Yes 1 | No | I don't know. |

Total: _____

b. To be completed by husband/male partner

Am I from a small family (1 or 2 children) or am I the only child?
.... Yes 1 | No | I don't know. |
Did I enter puberty late? .... Yes 2 | No | I don't know. |
Was any congenital abnormality ever mentioned? .... Yes 1 | No | I don't know. |
Do I not have to shave every day? .... Yes 1 | No | I don't know. |
Are my testes small and soft? (<15cm³) .... Yes 3 | No | I don't know. |
Is one of my testes in the inguinal canal or missing? .. Yes 3 | No | I don't know. |
Was I sexually active without a condom? .... Yes 2 | No | I don't know. |
Did I have a genital-tract infection, treated or untreated? . Yes 2 | No | I don't know. |
Did any of my previous partners develop genital-tract infections while with me?
.... Yes 2 | No | I don't know. |
Was I with someone for a long time and, despite of irregular use of birth control,
no pregnancy occurred?........................ Yes 2 | No | I don't know. |
Did any pregnancy from me end with an abortion or delivery that was followed
by significant changes in her menstrual flow quantity, pattern, color, and/or
interval or associated pain and PMS? .... Yes 3 | No | I don't know. |
Did anybody getting pregnant from me carry a complicated pregnancy
and/or give birth to a sickly child?................. Yes 3 | No | I don't know. |
Did a previous partner of mine develop allergies, asthma, uncontrolled weight
gain, and/or a thyroid problem following a previous delivery or abortion?
.... Yes 2 | No | I don't know. |
Did a previous partner of mine suffer from an unduly long postpartum/
abortion depression?........................... Yes 1 | No | I don't know. |
Did she need psychiatric therapy after such an event?. Yes 1 | No | I don't know. |
Did any previous relationship break up because my partner could not control her
moods/feelings/responses following an abortion/delivery?
.... Yes 1 | No | I don't know. |
Did she lose interest in sex after such an event? ...... Yes 1 | No | I don't know. |
Did she become alienated from me, children, parents, or friends after a pregnancy
related event?................................. Yes 1 | No | I don't know. |
Did I have an intervening chronic illness? .... Yes 1 | No | I don't know. |
Any hospital stays, with or without surgery? .... Yes 1 | No | I don't know. |
Any major surgery with catheterization of the bladder?.. Yes 1 | No | I don't know. |
Any surgical procedure on urethra, prostate, bladder? Cystoscopy?
.... Yes 1 | No | I don't know. |
Any surgery to correct congenital genito-urinary tract abnormality?
.... Yes 2 | No | I don't know. |
Did the quantity of the ejaculation or did my feelings change during
ejaculation?................................... Yes 2 | No | I don't know. |
Did I abuse drugs, alcohol, or nicotine? .... Yes 1 | No | I don't know. |
Did I use anabolic steroids for a long period of time? . Yes 1 | No | I don't know. |
Was I excessively obese before or ever after puberty?.. Yes 2 | No | I don't know. |
Am I on any drugs for the treatment of a chronic condition? (antibiotics, insulin,
CNS depressant, thyroid medication, anti-hypertensive, heart medication, ulcer
medication, colitis medication, steroids, or chemotherapy?
.... Yes 2 | No | I don't know. |

Total: _____

2. General Health Histories: You and Your Partner

a. To be completed by wife/female partner

Have I ever experienced: Heart disease? . . . . Yes 4 | No | I don't know. |
Hypertension? . . . . Yes 4 | No | I don't know. |
Cancer? . . . . Yes 4 | No | I don't know. |
Diabetes? . . . . Yes 4 | No | I don't know. |
Arthritis? . . . . Yes 1 | No | I don't know. |
Ulcer/Colitis? . . . . Yes 1 | No | I don't know. |
Cholecystitis/Gallstone? . . . . Yes 2 | No | I don't know. |
Kidney stone? . . . . Yes 3 | No | I don't know. |
Kidney infection? . . . . Yes 3 | No | I don't know. |
Asthma? . . . . Yes 2 | No | I don't know. |
Thyroid condition? . . . . Yes 1 | No | I don't know. |
Abnormal Pap smear? . . . . Yes 2 | No | I don't know. |
Chronic vaginitis/cystitis? . . . . Yes 2 | No | I don't know. |
Pelvic Inflammatory Disease? . . . . Yes 4 | No | I don't know. |
Endometriosis? . . . . Yes 2 | No | I don't know. |
Polycystic ovarian disease? . . . . Yes 3 | No | I don't know. |
Amenorrhea? . . . . Yes 2 | No | I don't know. |
Cervical cancer? . . . . Yes 2 | No | I don't know. |
Uterine/Ovarian cancer? . . . . Yes 4 | No | I don't know. |

Total: _____

b. To be completed by husband/male partner

Have I ever experienced: Heart disease?............. Yes 4 | No | I don't know. |
Hypertension? .... Yes 4 | No | I don't know. |
Cancer? .... Yes 4 | No | I don't know. |
Diabetes?....................................... Yes 4 | No | I don't know. |
Arthritis?....................................... Yes 1 | No | I don't know. |
Ulcer/Colitis? .... Yes 1 | No | I don't know. |
Cholecystitis/Gallstone? .... Yes 1 | No | I don't know. |
Kidney stone?.................................. Yes 3 | No | I don't know. |
Kidney infection?............................... Yes 3 | No | I don't know. |
Asthma? .... Yes 2 | No | I don't know. |
Thyroid condition? .... Yes 1 | No | I don't know. |
Congenital hernia?.............................. Yes 3 | No | I don't know. |
Undescended testes?............................ Yes 3 | No | I don't know. |
Varicocele? .... Yes 2 | No | I don't know. |
Non-specific Urethritis? .... Yes 3 | No | I don't know. |
Prostatitis?..................................... Yes 3 | No | I don't know. |
Epididymitis?................................... Yes 3 | No | I don't know. |
Orchitis? .... Yes 3 | No | I don't know. |
Bladder/Testis/Prostate cancer?................... Yes 4 | No | I don't know. |

Total: _____

3. Reproductive Health and Fertility Histories: You, Your Partner, and Parents

a. To be completed by wife/female partner

Did it take my parents a long time to produce their first child?
.... Yes 1 | No | I don't know. |
Did my parents experience:
  Any miscarriages? .... Yes 1 | No | I don't know. |
  Ectopic pregnancies? .... Yes 1 | No | I don't know. |
  Secondary infertility?........................... Yes 2 | No | I don't know. |
Was I born:
  Before or after a miscarriage or ectopic pregnancy? . Yes 3 | No | I don't know. |
  Prematurely? (>4wks) .... Yes 3 | No | I don't know. |
  Two weeks early or two weeks late?............... Yes 2 | No | I don't know. |
  Through cesarean section? .... Yes 1 | No | I don't know. |
During her pregnancy with me, did my mother experience:
  Premature labor? .... Yes 2 | No | I don't know. |
  High blood pressure/ preeclampsia?............... Yes 3 | No | I don't know. |
  Cervical incompetence?.......................... Yes 1 | No | I don't know. |
  Placental previa?................................ Yes 1 | No | I don't know. |
  Intrauterine growth retardation?................. Yes 2 | No | I don't know. |
Was I born with:
  Fetal distress? .... Yes 1 | No | I don't know. |
  Meconium? .... Yes 1 | No | I don't know. |
  Neonatal infections?............................ Yes 1 | No | I don't know. |
  Hyperbilirubinemia? .... Yes 1 | No | I don't know. |
As an infant, did I have:
  Asthma?.. Yes 2 | No | I don't know. |
  Colic? .... Yes 1 | No | I don't know. |
  Ear infections?................................. Yes 1 | No | I don't know. |
  Chronic tonsillitis? .... Yes 1 | No | I don't know. |
  Hernia?.. Yes 3 | No | I don't know. |
Did my mother experience postpartum depression? .. Yes 1 | No | I don't know. |

Total: _____

b. To be completed by husband/male partner

Did it take my parents a long time to produce their first child?
....Yes 1 | No | I don't know. |
Did my parents experience:
   Any miscarriages? ....Yes 1 | No | I don't know. |
   Ectopic pregnancies? ....Yes 1 | No | I don't know. |
   Secondary infertility?...........................Yes 2 | No | I don't know. |
Was I born:
   Before or after a miscarriage or ectopic pregnancy? . Yes 3 | No | I don't know. |
   Prematurely? (>4wks) ....Yes 3 | No | I don't know. |
   Two weeks early or two weeks late?...............Yes 2 | No | I don't know. |
   Through cesarean section? ....Yes 1 | No | I don't know. |
During her pregnancy with me, did my mother experience:
   Premature labor? ....Yes 2 | No | I don't know. |
   High blood pressure/ preeclampsia?..............Yes 3 | No | I don't know. |
   Cervical incompetence?.........................Yes 1 | No | I don't know. |
   Placental previa?...............................Yes 1 | No | I don't know. |
   Intrauterine growth retardation?..................Yes 2 | No | I don't know. |
Was I born with:
   Fetal distress? ....Yes 1 | No | I don't know. |
   Meconium? ....Yes 1 | No | I don't know. |
   Neonatal infections?............................Yes 1 | No | I don't know. |
   Hyperbilirubinemia? ....Yes 1 | No | I don't know. |
As an infant, did I have:
   Asthma?.......................................Yes 2 | No | I don't know. |
   Colic? ....Yes 1 | No | I don't know. |
   Ear infections?.................................Yes 1 | No | I don't know. |
   Chronic tonsillitis? ....Yes 1 | No | I don't know. |
   Hernia?..Yes 3 | No | I don't know. |
Did my mother experience postpartum depression? .. Yes 1 | No | I don't know. |

Total: _____

4. Reproductive Health and Fertility Histories: Siblings

a. To be completed by wife/female partner

Did any of my sisters/brothers experience any infertility problems?
(Miscarriages, ectopic pregnancies, etc.) . . . . Yes 1 | No | I don't know. |
Did it take my sister/brother a long time to produce their first child?
. . . . Yes 1 | No | I don't know. |
Did my siblings experience:
  Any miscarriages? . . . . Yes 1 | No | I don't know. |
  Ectopic pregnancies? . . . . Yes 1 | No | I don't know. |
  Secondary infertility? . . . . Yes 2 | No | I don't know. |
Were any of my nieces/nephews born:
  Before or after a miscarriage or ectopic pregnancy? . . Yes 3 | No | I don't know. |
  Prematurely? (>4wks) . . . . Yes 3 | No | I don't know. |
  Two weeks early or two weeks late? . . . . Yes 2 | No | I don't know. |
  Through cesarean section? . . . . Yes 1 | No | I don't know. |
During her pregnancy, did my sister/sister-in-law experience:
  Premature labor? . . . . Yes 2 | No | I don't know. |
  High blood pressure/ preeclampsia? . . . . Yes 3 | No | I don't know. |
  Cervical incompetence? . . . . Yes 1 | No | I don't know. |
  Placental previa? . . . . Yes 1 | No | I don't know. |
  Intrauterine growth retardation? . . . . Yes 2 | No | I don't know. |
Were any of my nieces/nephews born with:
  Fetal distress? . . . . Yes 1 | No | I don't know. |
  Meconium? . . . . Yes 1 | No | I don't know. |
  Neonatal infections? . . . . Yes 1 | No | I don't know. |
  Hyperbilirubinemia? . . . . Yes 1 | No | I don't know. |
As infants, did they have:
  Asthma? . . . . Yes 2 | No | I don't know. |
  Colic? . . . . Yes 1 | No | I don't know. |
  Ear infections? . . . . Yes 1 | No | I don't know. |
  Chronic tonsillitis? . . . . Yes 1 | No | I don't know. |
  Hernia? . . . . Yes 3 | No | I don't know. |
Did my sister-in-law experience postpartum depression?
. . . . Yes 1 | No | I don't know. |

Total: _____

b. To be completed by husband/male partner

Did any of my sisters/brothers experience any infertility problems?
(Miscarriages, ectopic pregnancies, etc.) . . . . Yes 1 | No | I don't know. |
Did it take my sister/brother a long time to produce their first child?
. . . . Yes 1 | No | I don't know. |
Did my siblings experience:
  Any miscarriages? . . . . Yes 1 | No | I don't know. |
  Ectopic pregnancies? . . . . Yes 1 | No | I don't know. |
  Secondary infertility? . . . . Yes 2 | No | I don't know. |
Were any of my nieces/nephews born:
  Before or after a miscarriage or ectopic pregnancy? . . Yes 3 | No | I don't know. |
  Prematurely? (>4wks) . . . . Yes 3 | No | I don't know. |
  Two weeks early or two weeks late? . . . . Yes 2 | No | I don't know. |
  Through cesarean section? . . . . Yes 1 | No | I don't know. |
During her pregnancy, did my sister/sister-in-law experience:
  Premature labor? . . . . Yes 2 | No | I don't know. |
  High blood pressure/ preeclampsia? . . . . Yes 3 | No | I don't know. |
  Cervical incompetence? . . . . Yes 1 | No | I don't know. |
  Placental previa? . . . . Yes 1 | No | I don't know. |
  Intrauterine growth retardation? . . . . Yes 2 | No | I don't know. |
Were any of my nieces/nephews born with:
  Fetal distress? . . . . Yes 1 | No | I don't know. |
  Meconium? . . . . Yes 1 | No | I don't know. |
  Neonatal infections? . . . . Yes 1 | No | I don't know. |
  Hyperbilirubinemia? . . . . Yes 1 | No | I don't know. |
As infants, did they have:
  Asthma? . . . . Yes 2 | No | I don't know. |
  Colic? . . . . Yes 1 | No | I don't know. |
  Ear infections? . . . . Yes 1 | No | I don't know. |
  Chronic tonsillitis? . . . . Yes 1 | No | I don't know. |
  Hernia? . . . . Yes 3 | No | I don't know. |
Did my sister-in-law experience postpartum depression?
. . . . Yes 1 | No | I don't know. |

Total: _____

5. GENERAL HEALTH HISTORIES: PARENTS
----

a. To be completed by wife/female partner

Mother:

Did my mother die before age 60 of any of the following diseases:
    Hypertension, Heart disease, Diabetes, Cancer?..... Yes 3 | No | I don't know. |
    Uterine/Ovarian cancer? .... Yes 4 | No | I don't know. |
If no, has she suffered from any of the following:
    Heart disease?................................. Yes 2 | No | I don't know. |
    Hypertension?................................. Yes 2 | No | I don't know. |
    Diabetes? .... Yes 2 | No | I don't know. |
    Cancer?.. Yes 2 | No | I don't know. |
    Ovarian/Uterine cancer? .... Yes 3 | No | I don't know. |
Did any my mother's brothers/sisters experience any of the above diseases?
    .... Yes 1 | No | I don't know. |

Father:

Did my father die before age 60 of any of the following diseases:
    Hypertension, Heart disease, Diabetes, Cancer?..... Yes 3 | No | I don't know. |
    Prostate/Bladder Cancer .... Yes 4 | No | I don't know. |
If no, has he suffered from any of the following:
    Heart disease?................................. Yes 2 | No | I don't know. |
    Hypertension?................................. Yes 2 | No | I don't know. |
    Diabetes? .... Yes 2 | No | I don't know. |
    Cancer?.. Yes 2 | No | I don't know. |
    Prostate/Bladder Cancer? .... Yes 3 | No | I don't know. |
Did any my father's brothers/sisters experience any of the above disease?
    .... Yes 1 | No | I don't know. |

Total: _____

b. To be completed by husband/male partner

Mother:

Did my mother die before age 60 of any of the following diseases:
    Hypertension, Heart disease, Diabetes, Cancer?..... Yes 3 | No | I don't know. |
    Uterine/Ovarian cancer? .... Yes 4 | No | I don't know. |
If no, has she suffered from any of the following:
    Heart disease?................................ Yes 2 | No | I don't know. |
    Hypertension?................................ Yes 2 | No | I don't know. |
    Diabetes? .... Yes 2 | No | I don't know. |
    Cancer?...................................... Yes 2 | No | I don't know. |
    Ovarian/Uterine cancer? .... Yes 3 | No | I don't know. |
Did any my mother's brothers/sisters experience any of the above diseases?
.... Yes 1 | No | I don't know. |

Father:

Did my father die before age 60 of any of the following diseases:
    Hypertension, Heart disease, Diabetes, Cancer?..... Yes 3 | No | I don't know. |
    Prostate/Bladder Cancer .... Yes 4 | No | I don't know. |
If no, has he suffered from any of the following:
    Heart disease?................................ Yes 2 | No | I don't know. |
    Hypertension?................................ Yes 2 | No | I don't know. |
    Diabetes? .... Yes 2 | No | I don't know. |
    Cancer?...................................... Yes 2 | No | I don't know. |
    Prostate/Bladder Cancer? .... Yes 3 | No | I don't know. |
Did any my father's brothers/sisters experience any of the above disease?
.... Yes 1 | No | I don't know. |

Total: _____

6. General Health Histories: Grandparents

a. To be completed by wife/female partner

Paternal Grandfather
Did my father's father die before age 60? .... Yes 1 | No | I don't know. |
If so, did he suffer from:
    Heart disease?................................. Yes 1 | No | I don't know. |
    Stroke? .... Yes 1 | No | I don't know. |
    Hypertension?................................. Yes 1 | No | I don't know. |
    Cancer?.. Yes 1 | No | I don't know. |
    Diabetes? .... Yes 1 | No | I don't know. |

Paternal Grandmother
Did my father's mother die before age 60? .... Yes 1 | No | I don't know. |
If so, did he suffer from:
    Heart disease?................................. Yes 1 | No | I don't know. |
    Stroke? .... Yes 1 | No | I don't know. |
    Hypertension?................................. Yes 1 | No | I don't know. |
    Cancer?.. Yes 1 | No | I don't know. |
    Diabetes? .... Yes 1 | No | I don't know. |

Maternal Grandfather
Did my mother's father die before age 60? .... Yes 1 | No | I don't know. |
If so, did he suffer from:
    Heart disease?................................. Yes 1 | No | I don't know. |
    Stroke? .... Yes 1 | No | I don't know. |
    Hypertension?................................. Yes 1 | No | I don't know. |
    Cancer?.. Yes 1 | No | I don't know. |
    Diabetes? .... Yes 1 | No | I don't know. |

Maternal Grandmother
Did my mother's mother die before age 60?.......... Yes 1 | No | I don't know. |
If so, did she suffer from:
    Heart disease?................................. Yes 1 | No | I don't know. |
    Stroke? .... Yes 1 | No | I don't know. |
    Hypertension?................................. Yes 1 | No | I don't know. |
    Cancer?.. Yes 1 | No | I don't know. |
    Diabetes? .... Yes 1 | No | I don't know. |

Total: _____

b. To be completed by husband/male partner

Paternal Grandfather
Did my father's father die before age 60? . . . . Yes 1 | No | I don't know. |
If so, did he suffer from:
    Heart disease?. . . . . Yes 1 | No | I don't know. |
    Stroke? . . . . Yes 1 | No | I don't know. |
    Hypertension?. . . . . Yes 1 | No | I don't know. |
    Cancer?. . . . . Yes 1 | No | I don't know. |
    Diabetes? . . . . Yes 1 | No | I don't know. |

Paternal Grandmother
Did my father's mother die before age 60? . . . . Yes 1 | No | I don't know. |
If so, did he suffer from:
    Heart disease?. . . . . Yes 1 | No | I don't know. |
    Stroke? . . . . Yes 1 | No | I don't know. |
    Hypertension?. . . . . Yes 1 | No | I don't know. |
    Cancer?. . . . . Yes 1 | No | I don't know. |
    Diabetes? . . . . Yes 1 | No | I don't know. |

Maternal Grandfather
Did my mother's father die before age 60? . . . . Yes 1 | No | I don't know. |
If so, did he suffer from:
    Heart disease?. . . . . Yes 1 | No | I don't know. |
    Stroke? . . . . Yes 1 | No | I don't know. |
    Hypertension?. . . . . Yes 1 | No | I don't know. |
    Cancer?. . . . . Yes 1 | No | I don't know. |
    Diabetes? . . . . Yes 1 | No | I don't know. |

Maternal Grandmother
Did my mother's mother die before age 60? . . . . Yes 1 | No | I don't know. |
If so, did she suffer from:
    Heart disease?. . . . . Yes 1 | No | I don't know. |
    Stroke? . . . . Yes 1 | No | I don't know. |
    Hypertension?. . . . . Yes 1 | No | I don't know. |
    Cancer?. . . . . Yes 1 | No | I don't know. |
    Diabetes? . . . . Yes 1 | No | I don't know. |

Total: _____

Glossary

Aerobic bacteria . . . . Bacteria that can live and grow in the presence of oxygen.

Anaerobic bacteria . . . A microorganism that thrives best or only in the absence of oxygen.

Androgen . . . A generic term for an agent, usually a hormone, e.g., testosterone or androsterone, that stimulates the activity of the accessory sex organs of the male, encourages the development of the male sex characteristics.

Anorexia. . . . . Diminished appetite, aversion to food.

Anovulatory ovary/anovulation. . . . . Suspension or cessation of ovulation.

Antibody. . . . .
A body or substance evoked by an antigen, and characterized by reaction specifically with the antigen in some demonstrable way—antibody and antigen each being defined in terms of the other. It is now supposed that antibodies may also exist naturally without being presents as a result of the stimulus provided by the introduction of an antigen.

Antigen. . . . .
Any of the various sorts of material, microorganisms, toxoids, exotoxins, foreign proteins, foreign cells or tissues and others that, as a result of coming in contact with appropriate tissues of an animal body, induces a state of sensitivity.

Aorta . . . A large artery of the elastic type, which is the main trunk of the systemic arterial system, arising from the base of the left ventricle.

ART . . . . Assisted reproductive technology.

Ascherman syndrome . . . .
Adhesions formed between the front and back walls of the uterus. Almost always secondary to an infection.

Aspartame/aspartame. . . . . A salt or ester of aspartic acid.

Autoimmune diseases/autoimmunity . . . .
Conditions in which antibodies are produced against the subject's own tissues.

Azospermic. . Absence of living or dead spermatozoa in the semen; failure of spermatogenesis.

Bulimia . . Morbidly increased appetite, often alternating with periods of anorexia.

Cervicitis . . Trachelitis; inflammation of the mucous membrane, frequently involving also the deeper structures of the cervix uteri.

Cervix . . . .
The lower part of the uterus extending from the isthmus of the uterus into the vagina.

Cesarean section . . . .
Surgical incision of the walls of the abdomen and uterus for delivery of offspring.

Chlamydia trachomatis . . . .
Spherical, nonmotile organisms that form compact intracytoplasmic microcolonies up to 10 um in diameter which (by division) give rise to infectious elementary bodies. Various strains of this species cause trachoma, inclusion conjunctivitis, lymphogranuloma venereum, pneumonia, nonspecific urethritis and PID.

Cholecystitis...............................Inflammation of the gallbladder.
Colic...............1) Related to the colon, 2) spasmodic pains in the abdomen.
Colposcopy........Examination of vagina and cervix by means of an endoscope.
Corpus luteum........................
The yellow endocrine body formed in the ovary in the site of a ruptured ovarian follicle. The life history of the corpus luteum begins immediately after ovulation. There is an early stage of proliferation or hyperemia and of vascularization before full maturity
Cystitis................................Inflammation of the urinary bladder.
Diabetes ....
Any of the various abnormal conditions characterized by the elevation of blood sugar and secretion and excretion of excessive amounts of urine.
Ectopic................................
Aberrant; heterotopic; out of place; a pregnancy occurring elsewhere than in the cavity of the uterus.
Ejaculation....................................Emission of seminal fluid.
Endocrinology............................
The science dealing with the internal secretions and their physiologic and pathologic relations.
Endometrial lining ....The lining of the endometrium.
Endometriosis...The ectopic occurrence of endometrial tissue, frequently forming cysts containing altered blood
Endometrium................................
The mucous membrane comprising the inner layer of the uterine wall; it consists of a simple, columnar epithelium and a lamina propria that contains simple tubular uterine glands.
Epididymis................................
The first, convoluted portion of the excretory duct of the testis, passing downward along the posterior border of this gland.
Estrogen ....
A generic term for any substance, whether naturally occurring or synthetic, that exerts biological effects characteristic of estrogenic hormones, such as estradiol; names for its ability to induce estrus in lower mammals. The ovary, placenta, testes and possible the adrenal cortex, as well as certain plants form estrogens.
Estrus ....
The portion or phase of the sexual cycle of female animals characterized by willingness to permit coitus.
Fallopian tubes ....
Either of the pair of tubes conducting the egg from the ovary to the uterus.
Fibroid ....
A benign uterine tumor resembling or composed of fibrous and muscular tissue.
Gamete ....Any germ cell, whether ovum or spermatozoon.
Gametogenesis...........The process of formation and development of gametes.
Giemsa technique...A staining technique originally introduced for demonstrating Negri bodies, the malarial organisms, spirochetes and protozoa and for differential staining of blood smears.
Gustav Giemsa ....A Hamburg bacteriologist. 1867-1948

Gonad . . . . . An organ that produces sex cells: the testis of a male or the ovary of a female.

Gonorrhea . . Catarrhal inflammation of the genital mucous membrane, caused by the bacterium Neisseria gonorrhea and transmitted chiefly by coitus.

Gram technique . . . . A method of differential staining of bacteria.

Hans C.J. Gram . . . . Danish bacteriologist.

Hormone . . . . , ...
A chemical substance formed and carried in the blood to another organ or part. Depending on the specificity of their effects, hormones can alter the functional activity and sometimes the structure of just one organ or of various numbers of them.

Hypogonadism . . . . Inadequate gonadal function, as manifested by deficiencies in gametogenesis and/or the secretion of gonadal hormones.

Idiopathic . . . . Particular to the individual, unknown cause.

Immunology . . . .
The science dealing with the various phenomena of immunity (antigen-antibody reactions).

Impotence . . . .
Lack of power in the male to copulate; may involve inability to achieve penile erection or to achieve ejaculation, or both; a manifestation, usually of a neurological or emotional dysfunction.

In vitro fertilization . . . . Test tube conception.

Induced labor . . . . To bring about the labor process .

Infertility, infertile . . . . Not fertile or productive.

Intratubal insemination . . . . Injection sperm into the fallopian tubes.

Intrauterine insemination . . . . Injecting sperm into the uterus.

Luteal . . . . Relating to the corpus luteum.

Lymphoma . . . .
A general term that includes various abnormally proliferative, neoplastic diseases of the lymphoid tissues.

Menometrorrhagia . . . .
Irregular or excessive bleeding during menstruation and between menstrual periods; this is a symptom, but not an acceptable diagnosis.

Menopause . . . .
Permanent cessation of the menses; termination of the menstrual life.

Menstruation . . . .
The periodic discharged of a bloody fluid from the uterus. Shedding of the uterine lining.

Morphology . . . . Detailed analysis of the sperm structure

Mycoplasma . . . . A genus of aerobic to facultatively anaerobic bacteria (family Mycoplasmataceae) containing Gram-negative cells, which do not possess a true cell wall. These organisms are found in humans and other animals and are parasitic to pathogenic.

Oligospermia . . . . A subnormal concentration of spermatozoa in the ejaculate.

Orchitis . . . . Inflammation of the testes.

Ovulation . . . . The release of an ovum from the ovarian follicle.

Pap test . . . .
A smear test from specimens from the cervix used to determine cancerous changes. Invented by George N. Papanicolaou.

Pathogen . . . . Any virus, microorganism, or other substance causing disease.

Pitocin . . . .
    A hormone like substance used to stimulate uterine contractions to induce or
    augment labor.
Polycystic . . . . . Composed of many cysts. Ovaries with several immature follicles.
Postcoital . . . . The time immediately after coitus.
Preeclampsia . . . .
    The development of hypertension with proteinuria or edema, or both due to
    pregnancy or the influence of a recent pregnancy.
Progesterone . . . . Corpus luteum hormone.
Prostate/prostata . . . . A chestnut-shaped body that surrounds the beginning of the
    urethra in the male; it consists of two lateral lobes that are connected anterior-
    ly by the isthmus and posteriorly by the middle lobe lying above and
    between the ejaculatory ducts. The secretion of the glands is a milky fluid that
    is discharged into the urethra at the time of ejaculation.
Prostatitis . . . . Inflammation of the prostate gland.
Scrotum . . . . A musculocutaneous sac containing the testes.
Syphilis . . An acute and chronic infectious disease caused by Treponema pallidum
    (Spirochaeta pallida) and transmitted by direct contact, usually through sexu-
    al intercourse.
Testis . . One of the two male reproductive glands, located in the cavity of the scro-
    tum.
Urethra . . . . A canal leading from the bladder, discharging the urine externally.
Uterus . . . .
    The womb; the hollow muscular organ in which the impregnated ovum is
    developed into the child.
Varicocele . . . . Enlargement of the veins of the spermatic cord, causing a boggy
    enlargement of the scrotum.
Vas deferens . . . .
    The ducts connecting the testes to the ejaculatory duct and ultimately to the
    urethra.
Vertical transmission . . . . Bacteria contamination acquired prior to or during birth.
Vesiculitis . . . Inflammation of any vesicle, specifically inflammation of the seminal
    vesicle.
Virus . . . . a term for a group of microbes which with few exceptions are capable of
    passing through fine filters that retain bacteria; they are incapable of growth
    or reproduction apart from living cells.

Index

Surgery, 64
Ovaries
Adhesions, consequences of, 25, 145
Biopsy, 44, 91
Cancer, 137
Congenitally depleted, 42
Damaged ovaries, 70
Diminished ovarian reserve, 84
Estradiol, diminished supply, 66, 127, 129
Estrogen production, 66, 71, 127
Follicles, this index
Formation of eggs, commencement and cessation, 58, 127
Location and function, 28, 54–55
Oophoritis, 61, 104
Ova and ovum, defined, 55
Ovarian Cyst, this index
Ovarian hormone deficiency, 25, 29, 66, 127
Paradox ovulation, 69–70, 132
Partial antibiotic therapy, 29
Peri-oophoritis, 104
Polycystic Ovarian Disease, this index
Premature ovarian failure, 92–93
Progesterone production, 66, 119, 127
Prolactin production, 127–128
Quality of eggs, 127
Runaway follicles, 127
Rushing out eggs, 128
Scarring of ovaries, 9
Secondary ovarian failure, 109
Senescence (aging), 127–128
Sugar-coated, 104
Surgery, 146
Unprotected intercourse depleting ovarian reserve, 108
Overview Of Fertility/Infertility
Generally, 53
Causes of Infertility, this index
Conception, pregnancy, and birth, 59–60
Ovulation
Generally, 28
Abnormal, generally, 9, 65–66
Bloating stomach after, 35
Clomid boost, 117
Congenitally depleted ovaries, 42

Exercise, effect of, 14
Luteal phase defect, 9, 25, 117, 131
Paradox ovulation, 69–70, 132
Pituitary hormones initiating, 57
Runaway eggs, 127
Rushing out eggs (multiple ovulations), 128, 131
Stress, effect of, 172
Ovulatory Mucus-Sperm Slide Test (OMSST)
Generally, 88
Ovum
Defined, 55

P
Paradox ovulation
Generally, 69–70, 132
Parasites
Diagnostic process, generally, 105–106
Treatment process, generally, 115–118
Trichomonads, this index
Parkinson's Disease
Pathogenic cause, 164
Paromomycin
Trichomonads therapy ineffective, 115
Pathogens
African-Americans statistics, 166
Asymptomatic, 11, 37
Cause of non-fertility serious illnesses, 5, 12, 13, 40, 44
Defined, 4, 25
Diagnostic process, generally, 83–86, 89
Explanation for infertility, 6, 8, 10, 11, 13, 44, 108, 160
Global trends, 166
Resistant bacterial strains, 162–163
Sensitivity report, 111
Tracking down evidence of pathogenic infection, 24–25, 44
Transmission of Pathogens, this index
Ways to safeguard your child's fertility in the future, 161–162
Pelvic Inflammatory Disease (PID)
Generally, 61–62
Chlamydia symptom, 90, 93

Number of sexual partners, likeli-
hood of genital tract contamina-
tion, 27
Pelvic inflammatory disease (PID),
27, 61
Polycystic ovarian syndrome (POS),
66–67
Sperm cell structure, 78
Transmission of infection greater
with high sperm count, 31
Trichomonas vaginalis, 105, 106
Unexplained infertility cases, 61, 73
Varicocele, 147–148
Woman's age, statistics on giving
birth and infertility, 4, 128, 135
**Statistics Involving Infection-Driven
Non-Infertility Illnesses**
Generally, 11–12
Family health history, 13
Stem Cell Research
General discussion, 168
Stenosis
Surgery for, 144
Stillbirth. See Fetal Demise or Stillbirth
Stomach Cancer
Pathogens as cause of, 5
Streptococcus
Aerobic bacteria, 96–101
Anaerobic bacteria, 101, 105
Group B Streptococcus, this index
Streptococcus Constellatus
Generally, 101, 105
Stress Management
Effect on conception and pregnancy,
17–19, 171–172
Exercise as means, 14
Pituitary gland's signals to ovaries,
66
Stroke
Pathogenic cause, 164
Submucosal Myomas
Operating on, 145
Substance Abuse. See Alcohol and
Recreational Drugs
Sugar-Coated Ovaries
Anaerobic infection, 104
Sulfarmethoxazole
Impact on reproductive functioning,
14–15
Surgery

Causing damage to reproductive
system, 10, 11, 71, 75
Endometriosis, 105
Extensive adhesions or large ovarian
cysts, 64
Female infertility, generally, 144–146
Hydrocele, 148
Hymen perforation, 71
Male infertility, generally, 147–150
Menometrorrhagia, 47
Ovaries, 70
Repeated adverse pregnancy out-
comes, surgical correction
advised, 71
Undescended testes, 76
Varicocele correction, 74, 147–148
Surrogacy
General discussion, 151–152
Syphilis
Babies getting, 41
Sexually transmitted disease (STD),
generally, 27

T

T Cells
Generally, 72
T-Shaped Uterus
Generally, 71
Mycoplasma infection, 95
Talks With Children About Sex
General discussion, 161–162
Testes
Congenitally depleted testes, 42, 76,
148
Inflammation as cause of infertility,
10
Location and function, 55, 57–58, 76,
148
Surgical removal, 148
Undescended, 76, 148
Testicles
Anatomy explained, 57
Diagram, 55
Hydrocele, 148
Hypothermia device, 148–149
Infection vertically transmitted, 43
Inguinal hernia, 76, 148
Varicocele, 10, 74, 147–148
Vas Deferens, this index
Testicular Biopsy

U

Printed in the United States
94838LV00001B/290/A